LIVING WELL WITH

Anxiety

Also by Carolyn Chambers Clark

Living Well with Menopause

The American Holistic Nurses' Association Guide to
Common Chronic Conditions: Self-Care Options
to Complement Your Doctor's Advice

Group Leadership Skills

Health Promotion in Communities:
Holistic and Wellness Approaches

Enhancing Wellness: A Guide for Self-Care

LIVING WELL WITH

Anxiety

What Your Doctor

Doesn't Tell You . . .

That You Need to Know

CAROLYN CHAMBERS CLARK, ARNP, Ed.D.

Founder of the Wellness Institute

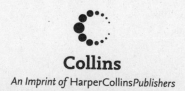

Collins
An Imprint of HarperCollins*Publishers*

HarperCollins books may be purchased for educational, business, or sales promotional use. For information please write: Special Markets Department, HarperCollins Publishers Inc., 10 East 53rd Street, New York, NY 10022.

FIRST EDITION

Designed by Joy O'Meara

Printed on acid-free paper

Library of Congress Cataloging-in-Publication Data

Clark, Carolyn Chambers.
    Living well with anxiety : what your doctor doesn't tell you—that you need to know / Carolyn Chambers Clark.
        p. cm.
    Includes bibliographical references and index.
    ISBN-10: 0-06-082377-1
    ISBN-13: 978-0-06-082377-1
    1. Anxiety—Popular works.   2. Anxiety—Alternative treatment—Popular works.   I. Title.

RC531.C53   2006
616.85'22—dc22
                                                        2005050399

03   04   05   06   07   WBC/RRD   10   9   8   7   6   5   4   3   2   1

MEDICAL DISCLAIMER

ACKNOWLEDGMENTS

I want once again to thank my husband, Anthony Auriemma. Without his love, terrific sense of humor, and ongoing support, this book would not have been possible.

I want to thank Lisa Shea, founder of BellaOnline, the largest source of information for women and families on the Internet. She gave me a chance to become an editor at http://HolisticHealth. bellaonline.com. That experience has enriched my life beyond my wildest dreams. It has allowed me to post articles and lead a forum from a holistic viewpoint, as well as offer a weekly newsletter updating my subscribers about new information about anxiety and related mental, physical, and spiritual topics.

Without my agent, Bob Diforio of the D4EO Literary Agency, this book would never have come to fruition. He found a home for my wellness writings at HarperCollins and was instrumental in obtaining a contract for this book in record time. Thank you, Bob, for your help, confidence, and wisdom.

Thanks to my editor at HarperCollins, Sarah Durand, who not only guided the direction of this book but made working on it a joy. I am bathed in a wonderful feeling of well-being knowing yet another of my books has found a home with a publisher who values a wellness and holistic approach.

A special thanks to all the clients over the years who have asked the important questions and shared what worked for them when dealing with the often confusing and sometimes overwhelming aspects of anxiety. Their stories inspired me to write this book.

CONTENTS

LIVING WELL WITH

Anxiety

Introduction

Anxiety conditions are the number-one mental health problem among American women and are second only to alcohol and drug abuse among men. The frequency of anxiety is also increasing among children, and it contributes to decreased social connectedness (divorce, living alone, decreased birthrate, marriage later in life). Increases in physical or psychological threats (violent crime, worry about nuclear war, fear of diseases such as AIDS, and the entrance of more women into the workforce) are identified as significant factors in the upswing of anxiety.

Approximately 10 percent of the population of the United States, or more than 30 million people, suffer from anxiety disorders each year, yet only a small proportion receive treatment. Many who suffer from high anxiety are too embarrassed or ashamed to discuss their anxieties. For many people, this book may provide the only help they will ever receive.

Let's take a look at some of the varied conditions that result from uncontrolled anxiety.

Hillary wakes up every night a couple of hours after going to sleep, her heart racing, feeling dizzy, with a tightness in her throat, and fearful something terrible is going to happen.

Joe just got a promotion because of his Internet sales ability. Now he must contribute to group sales meetings and he knows he's going to be tongue-tied, stammer instead of speak coherently, and get so restless he won't be able to sit still.

Ruth, a bank teller, has been forcing herself to go to work, and once she gets there, she's afraid she might say or do something silly, and want to leave.

Adam just entered college, and he's afraid to speak up in class, even though he knows the answer, and he freezes when he has to take a written exam.

Sylvia was raped a year ago. She continues to have repetitive distressing thoughts about the event, as well as nightmares, flashbacks, and emotional numbness.

▌ Why Anxiety Is Such a Problem Today

Anxiety conditions appear as a result of cumulative stress over time. Individuals in Western societies experience more stress than ever before. As a result, they experience more anxiety. The increased pace of modern society, the increased rate of technological change, the relative absence of traditionally prescribed values, a barrage of inconsistent worldviews presented in the media, terrorism threats—these and other factors make it more difficult to remain calm and to experience a sense of stability or consistency in their lives. The result is increased stress and anxiety. As anxiety continues to mount in our society, this book can provide the comfort and specific direction anxious individuals need.

■ A Traditional Medical Approach May Not Be Enough

For most anxiety-related conditions, the best that medicine can do is keep some of your symptoms at bay, and even that claim is questionable. The more we learn about the medications used to treat anxiety, the more we learn that these drugs often have unwanted effects that are worse than the anxiety itself.

The root cause of anxiety is rarely—if ever—addressed in a medical model. Only the symptoms are treated. That means you may never learn the source of your anxiety, and, as you may have already discovered, fear of the unknown brings on the worst kind of anxiety.

You may be fearful your anxiety is untreatable, or that it means you are crazy, or on your way to a lifetime of hospitalization and treatment. You may be fearful your anxiety may build into dramatically worsening conditions and phobias. You may be fearful that even though you're learning to deal with your anxiety, you suspect that new symptoms will appear and you will be unable to control them. You may be fearful that for the most part, doctors, unless they are psychiatrists, think you're faking it, or that your problems are all in your head. You may be fearful because most doctors don't have an answer when you ask if your anxiety is going to affect your family, work, and friends. You may be fearful that, over time, your anxiety is going to lead to other, more dangerous, conditions such as heart attacks, suicide, or even cancer. You may be afraid that you will never be able to overcome your anxiety, that you cannot stop its inexorable march as it seems to envelop and overtake every facet of your life. You may be afraid that there are no answers, no cure, no respite from the discomfort you feel and that no one really understands what you're going through.

Rest assured, there are answers, and there are ways you can learn to reduce your anxiety.

You just aren't likely to hear them from the typical HMO or primary-care physician, who may not even recognize or diagnose your condition, much less know how to treat it, especially now that typical HMO appointments are mandated to end in fifteen minutes or less.

You may not be able to obtain an answer from the average psychiatrist, either. These doctors must rush through dozens of patients a day, prescribing drugs and monitoring their effects. They simply don't have the time, and sometimes don't have the know-how, to delve into the complicated and connected conditions anxiety evokes.

And even those medical doctors who consider themselves experts in treating anxiety rarely venture into the uncharted territory of dealing with the source of anxiety. Most are content to focus on treating the symptoms of anxiety, not the source. They are comfortable prescribing anti-anxiety drugs, but ask these doctors how to help you remove the source of your anxiety and they will probably draw a blank.

▋ Why I Wrote This Book

My master's degree is in psychiatric/mental-health nursing and my minor at the doctoral level was psychology. My major in my doctoral program was education—specifically, novel methods of teaching and learning. I am also board certified as an advanced holistic/wellness practitioner.

Over the years I've experienced high degrees of anxiety due to graduate school stress, performance anxiety (when I first started to make presentations to large audiences), a fear of heights (after I was almost pushed off a second-floor balcony), as well as the many stresses and strains of our society that create anxiety. As a result,

I've had to learn how to reduce my stress, and thereby my anxiety. I've also taught many of my clients wellness procedures I've developed for reducing stress and enhancing calm through my Wellness Institute workshops, my private clinical practice, and on my website, http://HolisticHealth.bellaonline.com.

A wellness approach to anxiety focuses not only on the mind but also on the body and spirit—the whole person. I've personally and professionally explored alternative and complementary methods for reducing anxiety, including cognitive-behavioral approaches, yoga, relaxation therapy, affirmations, coping skills, environmental changes, herbs, and nutrition. I wrote this book because anxiety pervades all our lives . . . and because you need to know how to reduce it if you want to live well.

Variations of my story are repeated every day when someone suffering from high anxiety wonders, as I did, if the panic I felt meant I was going crazy. Or when someone who is fearful of heights—or animals or elevators or airplanes or some other situation—questions if they will ever overcome their fear and learn to remain calm in previously upsetting situations.

▌ Why You May Need This Book

This book is for you if . . .

- you strongly suspect you are suffering from high anxiety but are having difficulty finding someone to explain to you what the condition is about.
- you aren't sure if your discomfort points to anxiety but you're trying to find out more.
- you've been diagnosed with an anxiety condition and been prescribed pills but want more information about your condition.

- you are receiving what your doctor thinks is sufficient treatment for your anxiety but you still don't feel well.
- you're an open-minded health practitioner looking for innovative ways to understand and help your patients who suffer from high anxiety.
- you want to learn about living well with anxiety from the perspective of an empowered consumer.

▌ About This Book

Living Well with Anxiety is different from most books on anxiety. This is *your* book, written by a nurse practitioner who has not only counseled individuals with anxiety conditions but has experienced high anxiety and has learned ways to reduce anxiety to manageable levels and teach them to you.

Living Well with Anxiety provides the type of information about anxiety you may not find out from a doctor, pharmaceutical company, patient organizations, or in other books about anxiety. In this book I talk honestly with you about the traditional medical approaches to anxiety, including the drugs that are prescribed for specific conditions and their risks. But this book is really about living with anxiety and the kinds of self-care measures you can take to reduce and manage it.

In this book, you'll find out things your doctor may not tell you about risks, diagnoses, drugs, and alternative approaches that work to reduce anxiety. You'll also hear the voices of real people just like you who have struggled with anxiety and learned to deal with health-care practitioners, tried different approaches, suffered setbacks, and enjoyed successes. Each person quoted in this book expressed a determination to share his or her own story, difficulties, ideas, advice, and hope with you. That's why you'll be able to recognize your own experiences, fears, and frustrations, and be touched and moved by the incredibly honest and direct stories of others who have learned to live well with anxiety. Above all, you'll know you are not alone in your struggle.

▌ My Disclaimer

I hope what you learn in this book will help you decide what kinds of health-care practitioner to seek, what questions to ask them, and what your goals are. Seek out caring, informed health-care practitioners and work in a partnership with them. Don't try to go this alone. Seek out the conventional, alternative, and complementary practitioners to be your partners in wellness. And don't forget to share this book with them.

PART ONE

Anxiety and Medical Treatment

1

Anxiety: Causes and Effects

Anxiety is frequently confused with other feelings, especially fear. You may call anxiety "nerves" or "nervousness," but that may be the only information you have about the condition.

■ What Is Anxiety?

The word *anxiety* has been used since the 1500s and comes from the Latin word *anxius*, which means worry of an unknown event. Worry then leads to a state of apprehension and uncertainty, which results in both physical and psychological effects.

Although you may not know the difference between anxiety and fear, the two terms refer to entirely different feelings. Fear is usually directed at an external danger. The event you fear is identifiable. You may fear stepping off a curb when a car is speeding by at sixty miles an hour, or when a neighbor's dog suddenly jumps out at you.

Anxiety has no such easily recognizable source and is often called an unexplained discomfort. You may have a sense of danger when experiencing anxiety, but the feeling is vague, and if asked, you may say your feeling is related to "something bad happening," or "losing control."

Anxiety has physical, emotional, mental, and even spiritual effects. Physical effects include shortness of breath, heart palpitations, trembling or shaking, sweating, choking, nausea or abdominal distress, hot flashes or chills, dizziness or unsteadiness. Because anxiety is so uncomfortable, you may convert your anxiety into anger or other feelings. Emotional effects include feelings such as worry, anger, panic, and terror. Mental effects include thinking you're going to die, or that you're going crazy or are out of control. Spiritual effects include alienation and feeling detached and out of touch with yourself and others.

▮ What Causes Anxiety?

Everyone experiences anxiety. It is what makes us more human than otherwise, to paraphrase Dr. Harry Stack Sullivan. This psychoanalyst created the Theory of Interpersonal Relations and taught that much mental suffering is a result of communication that is interfered with by anxiety. According to Sullivan, anxiety is a normal reaction to unmet needs and other stresses, such as disapproval (first from parents and then from oneself or others). Anxiety can also be viewed as a protective mechanism that keeps you safe from situations believed to be threatening.

Whether or not anxiety develops into a chronic condition that interferes with your life depends on your genes, your early family experiences, your ongoing stress (which can affect brain activity), medical conditions, toxins you encounter, and drugs and stimulants you take. Let's examine these in a little more detail.

1. **Your genes can contribute to anxiety conditions** if you are born a volatile, excitable, reactive type of person who is easily set off by

a threat. In this case, you may be especially prone to panic attacks, which are really just your body overreacting by pouring adrenaline out of your adrenal glands and into your bloodstream. This leads to a racing heart, shallow breathing, profuse sweating, trembling and shaking, and cold hands and feet as your body readies itself to either fight or flee. Since there is no real threat, you are left with the chemical reactions flooding your body. Luckily, the adrenaline released during panic tends to be reabsorbed by the liver and kidneys within a few minutes, and the attack subsides.

2. Childhood experiences can contribute to anxiety conditions if you had parents who were overly cautious or critical, if you were neglected, rejected, abandoned, incurred physical or sexual abuse, grew up in a family where one or both parents were alcoholic, or had parents who suppressed your expression of feelings and self-assertiveness.

Jeff, a kindergarten teacher, was sexually abused by his uncle, a pet store owner. Jeff didn't seem to have any anxiety problems until he turned nineteen, when he developed phobias about animals and heights. He stayed away from high places and animals and was able to complete college and start teaching. Gradually he became unable to leave his house or even his bedroom. He found a therapist who worked with him until he was able to leave his bedroom and eventually his house. He has returned to teaching but continues to see his therapist monthly as a preventive measure.

3. Cumulative stress over many years has also been implicated in the development of anxiety conditions, and a stressful lifestyle that avoids exercise, healthy nutrition, daily relaxation, social support, and self-nurturing activities can put you at increased risk. Years of heavy smoking often precede anxiety disorders, especially agoraphobia, generalized anxiety, and panic disorder. The connection appears to be impaired breathing ability. Your serotonin level may be involved, especially if you develop obsessive-compulsive traits. There is also a theory that reduced levels of gamma-aminobutyric acid (GABA) can contribute to generalized anxiety.

There are numerous medical conditions that can lead to increased anxiety or panic attacks. *Hyperventilation syndrome* is a condition in which you breathe in the upper part of your chest. This results in symptoms very much like panic attacks, including light-headedness, shortness of breath, dizziness, trembling, and/or tingling in your hands. *Hypoglycemia*, or low blood sugar level, also mimics the symptoms of panic. *Hyperthyroidism* (excess secretion of thyroid hormone) can lead to heart palpitations, insomnia, anxiety, and sweating that can add to your normal anxiety. *Mitral valve prolapse* (a harmless defect in the valve separating the upper and lower chambers of the heart that may cause the heart to beat out of rhythm) occurs more frequently in people who have panic attacks. *Premenstrual syndrome* (PMS) can worsen panic attacks. *Inner ear disturbances* can lead to dizziness, light-headedness, and unsteadiness, any of which can add to your anxiety.

Other situations that can set off or worsen anxiety or panic include taking stimulants (cocaine, amphetamines, caffeine, aspartame), high blood pressure, exposure to environmental toxins (pesticides, food additives, lead, chlorine, fluoride, or cadmium, for example), heart failure or irregular heart beats, clot in the lung, emphysema, deficiencies in vitamins or minerals, concussion, epilepsy, parathyroid disease, Cushing's syndrome, thyrotoxicosis, and withdrawal from drugs (especially tranquilizers, sedatives, and alcohol).

Panic attacks or *phobias* (persistent and unreasonable fear that results in a strong desire to avoid a dreaded object, activity, or situation) can also be triggered by past traumatic situations.

■ The Learned Aspects of Anxiety

Learning to be anxious starts very early in life—in infancy, if not before. You learn to sense (or "pick up") worry when a parent signals disapproval with gestures such as frowning, tightening the lips or jaw, grimacing, or pointing fingers at you. Anxiety is a very uncomfortable feeling, and being around an anxious person can make you feel anxious, too. In this sense, anxiety is contagious.

As an infant, you learned what displeased or created anxiety in your parents, and as a result you fashioned your behavior, and maybe even your personality, to please them. You also acted in the way they approved because it reduced your anxiety—the calmer they were, the calmer you were. You learned the "good me" (what your parents approved of), the "bad me" (what your parents disapproved of), and the "not me" (aspects of living so dreadful or horrifying, at least according to your parents, that they may be dissociated and not remembered in adulthood, even when someone else points them out).

According to Harry Stack Sullivan, a feeling of anxiety is most apt to occur in situations in which your dignity and prestige are threatened by other people, and from which you are unable to escape. This includes embarrassing or unfamiliar settings.

■ What Are the Effects of Anxiety?

There are varying degrees of anxiety. Your ability to function is dependent on the level of discomfort you experience.

Mild anxiety can be a good thing. Without it, you'd be constantly drifting off to sleep, probably couldn't hold a coherent discussion or achieve any of your goals. Mild anxiety is necessary for learning to take place. As mild anxiety increases, it can lead to sleeplessness, restlessness, hostility, belittling, and misunderstandings.

As anxiety increases, your perception of what is going on around you decreases. Your hands or underarms may start to perspire, pulse and respiration increase, you may have "butterflies" in your stomach, diarrhea, frequent urination, tension headaches, fatigue, and/or increased muscle tension. You may speak more quickly, or more slowly, than usual.

When severe anxiety occurs, you start to pay attention only to parts of experiences and begin to block out the threat you feel. Learning does not occur at this level of anxiety, and your attention span is short. Your chances of understanding what is happening to you or of taking reasonable action are nil. You may focus on one small detail or on scattered details from many experiences. You may perspire profusely, and your pulse and blood pressure rise even higher. You may breathe rapidly in the upper part of your chest, and your lips and mouth may be quite dry. You may stammer, speak loudly, rapidly, in a high-pitched voice, or be hesitant. You may tremble, shiver, hold a rigid posture or clench your fists.

Panic is the most extreme level of anxiety. You may blow things way out of proportion, may experience terror and feelings of unreality and be unable to communicate with other people. Because the higher levels of anxiety are so distressing, you may convert your anxiety to anger, which can bring you back to feeling in control again, even though your anger is unreasonable. You can also convert your anxiety into withdrawal by calling in sick, canceling appointments, or retiring to bed. You may convert your anxiety into physical symptoms such as high blood pressure, tension headaches, diarrhea, fatigue, or other physical symptoms.

■ What Maintains Anxiety Conditions

Once you develop a specific way of thinking, feeling, and coping with anxiety, these behaviors can perpetuate anxiety. You can add to you feelings of discomfort by blaming the way you feel on some external happening or some other person. When you do that, you probably feel helpless because something outside of you is responsible for your anxiety. When you begin to take responsibility for your anxiety, you can begin to do something about it.

Much of this book is devoted to helping you learn new ways to cope with anxiety. Although many actions can keep an anxiety condition going, the following are the most common and are the easiest to change:

1. Avoidant Behaviors As long as you continue avoiding situations or objects that cause you anxiety, your anxiety will continue. Avoiding a situation doesn't eliminate it. You continue to worry and spend a great deal of energy to make sure you don't have to confront the situation or object. The key to unlearning your phobic reaction is to approach the upsetting situation or object in small steps. Imagery and desensitization are key to this effort and are discussed in chapter 9.

2. Negative Self-Talk We all talk to ourselves in our minds. Sometimes it's so automatic and subtle you don't notice it. Self-talk can be positive and encouraging or can be negative and create more anxiety. It is the following kinds of self-talk that must be silenced, including: "What if I have another panic attack?" "I'll never be able to deal with this!" "What if I lose control of myself?" "What will people think if I lose control?" "I'm having a heart attack—I just know it!" "My legs feel so weak, I can't walk." This kind of talking scares you even more and aggravates the physical aspects of anxiety. The good news is that you can learn to stop your negative self-talk and replace it with positive, encouraging messages. See chapter 9 for more information on this topic.

3. Mistaken Beliefs It is these mistaken beliefs that bring about negative self-talk. If you believe you are losing control, you can talk yourself and everyone else around you into believing that it's true. If you're programmed to believe life is meant to be hard, then you will think something is wrong when things go your way or people offer help. If you believe the world is a dangerous place and people can't be trusted, you will live a life filled with suspicion and will veer away from taking the risks necessary to overcome many anxiety conditions. See chapter 9 for more information on mistaken beliefs and how to overcome them.

4. Denial of Feelings When you deny anger, frustration, sadness, and even excitement, you can feel more anxious and not know why. You may have discovered that after you let out your anger or have a good cry, you feel more at ease, calmer. Expressing your feelings is a good way to reduce your anxiety.

5. Lack of Assertiveness Assertiveness is the vehicle that allows you to express your feelings in a respectful but honest way to other people. If you're not assertive, you may fuss and stew inwardly or avoid the person or the expression of how you feel. You may think it's not nice to be open about what you want and need because you might alienate the other person. The problem with not being assertive is that it builds resentment and confinement, two feelings that aggravate anxiety conditions. You can learn to be assertive. Find out more in chapter 10.

6. Muscle Tension When you feel uptight, you have tight muscles, and this restricts your breathing, healthy heartbeats, digestion, circulation, thought, and just about all body processes. You may have learned that when your body is tense, your mind races. When you relax your muscles, your mind will slow and calm. Anxiety cannot exist in a relaxed body, so the key is to use relaxation skills to be at peace. Vigorous exercise and deep muscle relaxation can help you remain calm. See chapters 8 and 9 for more information.

7. Lack of Self-Nurturing You may have a deep sense of insecurity due to a parent's neglect, abandonment, abuse, overprotection, negative criticism, alcoholism, or chemical dependency. Growing up in this kind of household means you never received consistent or reliable nurturing as a child and so you never learned how to take care of yourself in a loving and nurturant way. You probably feel anxious and overwhelmed by the adult demands placed upon you, and this can lead to perpetuating your anxiety condition. Learning to nurture your "inner child" is the way to grow and learn to be a responsible adult. See chapters 9 and 10 for more information.

8. Poor Nutrition Drinking lots of coffee and sodas, eating junk and fast foods, sugar, food additives, foods your body is sensitive to, and eating while doing something else can increase your anxiety. Just eliminating caffeine from your diet (including the caffeine in over-the-counter medicines) can relieve a great deal of anxiety and worry. See chapter 5 for more information.

9. Stressful Lifestyle Lack of time-management skills, not grieving losses and changes, burning the candle at both ends, smoking, drinking, and taking drugs can worsen your anxiety condition and even bring it on. See chapters 5–9 for more information on how to reduce your stress.

10. Lack of Meaning and Purpose We are all spiritual beings. If you've lost (or never developed) a sense of purpose for your life, something larger than immediate self-gratification, you will tend to be bored and anxious. See chapter 10 for ways to find meaning and purpose.

2

Self-Diagnosing Your Anxiety

If you want to learn more about your anxiety, charting your reactions in specific situations can be very helpful. Because anxiety is often unexplained discomfort, identifying what is happening right before, during, and after your anxious moments can help you decide what to do to reduce it. Use the Self-Diagnosis Checklist to determine when you have anxiety.

Self-Diagnosis Checklist

____ **1.** I feel uncomfortable and experience building tension or discomfort that seems to come out of the blue when I think about a particular situation.

____ **2.** I avoid specific situations that make me feel uncomfortable.

____ **3.** I have at least four of the following symptoms at the same time: shortness of breath or feeling smothered; heart palpitations (rapid or irregular heartbeat); trembling or shaking; choking; dizziness or unsteadiness; nausea or abdominal distress; numbness, feeling detached or out of touch with myself; fear of dying; fear of going crazy or out of control; hot flashes or chills; sweating without exertion.

___ **4.** I worry excessively, and so I feel restless, keyed up or on edge, irritable, easily fatigued, have trouble falling or staying asleep or I wake up tired, have tense and tight muscles, have difficulty concentrating, and/or find my mind going blank.

___ **5.** I have recurring intrusive thoughts such as hurting or harming a close relative, being contaminated by dirt or a toxic substance, fearing I forgot to lock my door or turn off an appliance, and/or have unpleasant fantasies of catastrophe.

___ **6.** I perform ritualistic actions such as washing my hands or counting to relieve my discomfort because I have fears that keep entering my mind.

___ **7.** I have witnessed or been subjected to a life-threatening experience and have persistent symptoms that have lasted for at least a month, including repetitive and distressing thoughts, nightmares, flashbacks, attempts to reenact the situation, emotional numbness (out of touch with your emotions—feeling no anger, sadness, guilt, or relief), feeling detached from other people, losing interest in activities that once gave me pleasure, sleep or concentration problems, startling easily, irritability and/or have outbursts of anger.

Key to Your Answers:

If you checked #1 (just thinking about a situation brings on discomfort), you have *anticipatory anxiety.*

If you checked #2 (your discomfort arises only in response to being in a specific situation), you have what is called *situational anxi-*

ety and you are likely dealing with *agoraphobia,* or fear of going to specific places or being alone. If your discomfort is related to being in social situations and is related to avoiding humiliating or embarrassing yourself, you may be suffering from a *social phobia.*

If you checked #3 and you include among your symptoms shortness of breath or feeling smothered, you have *panic attacks.* If your anxiety forces you to avoid certain situations, you have a *phobia.* If the avoidance is of places, such as driving on freeways, going to doctors, riding in elevators, using public transportation, going over bridges or going through tunnels, eating in restaurants, going to work, and so forth you are likely dealing with *agoraphobia.*

If you checked #4 you probably have a *generalized anxiety disorder.*

If you checked #5 you may have an *obsessive-compulsive disorder with obsessions only.*

If you checked #6 you are probably dealing with an *obsessive-compulsive disorder with both obsessions and compulsions.*

If you checked #7 you are probably in *post-traumatic stress* or *nonspecific anxiety condition.*

▋ How You Maintain Your Anxiety Disorder

As mentioned in the previous chapter, what you're doing to keep your symptoms going is crucial for you to identify so you can obtain relief.

Sarah, a thirty-two-year-old kindergarten teacher suffered from panic attacks and agoraphobia. By taking the Self-Diagnosis of Anxiety Maintenance Checklist (see below), she discovered that her actions, including negative self-talk, poor nutrition, and a negative lifestyle, added to her anxiety.

Complete the following checklist to find out how you might be maintaining your anxiety disorder by the things you do.

Self-Diagnosis of Anxiety Maintenance Checklist

Check the factors you think might be helping to maintain your anxiety. If you check an item, find the chapter in this book that will tell you more about how to overcome this behavior.

_____ **1.** Avoiding situations or objects that make me anxious. (chapter 9)

_____ **2.** Using negative self-talk. (chapter 9)

_____ **3.** Holding mistaken beliefs. (chapter 9)

_____ **4.** Not sharing my feelings. (chapters 9 and 10)

_____ **5.** Not being assertive. (chapter 10)

_____ **6.** Holding too much body tension. (chapters 8 and 9)

_____ **7.** Lack of self-nurturing skills. (chapters 9 and 10)

_____ **8.** Poor nutrition. (chapter 5)

_____ **9.** Leading a high-stress life. (chapter 7 and 8)

_____ **10.** Not having meaning or a sense of purpose to my life. (chapter 10)

Go back and pick three of the ten causes of anxiety and pledge to work on them daily for the next month. Write the word _pledge_ after each of the three. Work through the chapters that relate to your choices first, before reading the rest of this book.

3

Types of Anxiety Disorders

In the United States, anxiety disorders are the most commonly diagnosed mental condition of the adult population ages eighteen through fifty-four. Anxiety disorders cost more than $42 billion a year, almost one-third of the $148 billion total mental health bill. More than $22.84 billion of those costs are due to the repeated use of health-care services because anxiety disorders can mimic physical illnesses.

■ Diagnosing Your Condition

The first thing a physician will do is diagnose your anxiety to see if you have a disorder. Your practitioner will take a thorough history, keeping in mind that your chief complaint may not be anxiety at all. In fact, many individuals with anxiety disorders often have vague complaints such as diarrhea, insomnia, dizziness, or shortness of breath. They're not always sure what is causing the problem.

You will be asked questions about your feelings of anxiety, nervousness, fear, and depression. You may be asked whether similar symptoms have ever occurred in the past, what helped you to re-solve them, if you've tried those actions recently, and whether they help now.

Some questions you may be asked are: "What was the attitude toward drinking in your family?" or "Did your parents or grandpar-ents tend to drink when under pressure?" or "Did anyone in your family ever have problems with nerves, such as having a nervous breakdown?" or "How is your anxiety interfering with your life?"

Because many physical problems can lead to anxiety symptoms, your health-care practitioner will also try to rule out diseases of the heart, thyroid, kidney, nervous system, lung, and blood by doing a physical examination. You may also be asked about nutritional defi-ciencies (including lack of B-vitamins and iron) as well as what drugs you take, and how much alcohol you take, because they can also make you anxious.

▌ Generalized Anxiety Disorder (GAD)

Women are twice as likely as men to be afflicted with generalized anxiety disorder (GAD). One third of afflicted adults had their first symptoms in childhood. The essential characteristic of GAD is ex-cessive uncontrollable worry about everyday things. Everybody worries, but GAD is diagnosed when constant worry affects your ability to function in daily life for at least six months. GAD can oc-cur in combination with other anxiety disorders, depression, or sub-stance abuse. Physical symptoms include muscle tension, sweating, nausea, cold and clammy hands, difficulty swallowing, jumpiness, stomach and intestinal discomfort, and diarrhea. If you suffer from GAD, you tend to be irritable and complain about feeling on edge, you tire easily and have trouble sleeping. If you're in a relationship, GAD is apt to impact it negatively.

Because GAD lacks some of the dramatic symptoms of panic attacks or phobias, it may be difficult to diagnose. To make a diagnosis, your physician may ask you . . .

1. Do you worry excessively most days, and has this been happening for at least six months?
2. Do you worry unreasonably about work or school or your health?
3. Do you believe you can't control how much you worry?
4. Do you feel restless, keyed up, and on edge a lot of the time?
5. Do you tire easily?
6. Is it hard for you to concentrate?
7. Are you irritable?
8. Are your muscles tight and tense?
9. Do you have trouble falling asleep or staying asleep, or do you toss and turn and get up feeling tired?
10. Does your worry interfere with your daily life?

Will, a twenty-eight-year-old mechanic, was having trouble falling asleep. He tossed and turned and woke up feeling tired. He felt on edge a lot of the time and as a result got into arguments with the other mechanics; he had unreasonable worries about the work he was doing and didn't feel he had any control over his discomfort. Will's physician diagnosed him with generalized anxiety disorder and gave him a prescription for an anti-anxiety drug.

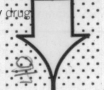

∎ Panic Disorder

About 3 million Americans, women more than men, are likely to be afflicted with panic disorder. A *panic attack* is defined as the abrupt onset of an episode of intense fear or discomfort that peaks in approximately ten minutes and includes at least four of the following symptoms: feeling of imminent danger or doom, need to escape, palpitations, sweating, trembling, shortness of breath or a smothering feeling, a feeling of choking, chest pain or discomfort, nausea or abdominal discomfort, dizziness or light-headedness, a sense of things seeming unreal (*depersonalization*), a fear of losing control or "going crazy," a fear of dying, tingling sensations, chills or hot flashes.

Three types of panic attack can be diagnosed. *Unexpected panic attacks* come "out of the blue" without warning and for no discernible reason. *Situational panic attacks* occur in specific situations, for example upon entering an elevator or a tunnel. *Situationally predisposed panic attacks* occur only sometimes in upsetting situations; for example, an individual may sometimes have a panic attack while driving, but not always. Many people diagnosed with panic attacks also suffer from major depression.

To be diagnosed with panic disorder, you must suffer at least two unexpected panic attacks, followed by at least one month of concern over having another attack. You may also be prone to situational panic attacks and worry about the physical and emotional consequences of your attacks. You may be convinced that the attacks you suffer indicate a serious illness and you will submit to frequent medical tests. Even after all the tests come back negative, you will probably remain worried that you do have a serious condition. You may even try to avoid the scene of a previous attack, hoping you can prevent another one.

The age of onset of panic disorder varies from adolescence to mid-thirties. Very few suffer from panic attacks in childhood.

Agoraphobia, or the fear of having a panic attack in a place from which you cannot escape, often coincides with panic disorder. You may refuse to leave your home, or develop a fixed "safe" route, such as between home and work, from which you cannot deviate. It may feel impossible to travel beyond what you consider your safety zone without suffering severe anxiety.

To diagnose your condition, your physician will probably ask you . . .

1. For no apparent reason do you have repeated, unexpected attacks during which you are overcome by intense fear or discomfort?

2. During this attack do you experience a pounding heart, sweating, trembling or shaking, shortness of breath, choking, chest pain, nausea or abdominal discomfort, "jelly" legs, dizziness, feelings of unreality or of being detached from yourself, fear of dying, numbness or tingling sensations, chills or hot flashes, or a fear of places you can't escape from?

3. For at least one month following an attack have you felt persistent concern about having another one, having a heart attack, or "going crazy," or have you changed your behavior so you won't have another attack?

4. Does having to travel without a companion trouble you?

▌ Obsessive-Compulsive Disorder (OCD)

OCD includes uncontrollable *obsessions*. These are recurring thoughts or impulses that are intrusive or inappropriate and cause you anxiety; for example, coming into contact with dirt, germs, or "unclean" objects, doubts about locking doors or turning off machines or appliances, extreme orderliness, or aggressive impulses or thoughts (such as to yell "fire" in a crowded theater).

Compulsions can also be involved. Compulsions are repetitive behaviors; for example, cleaning your house constantly, washing your hands repeatedly, or showering many times a day.

In both cases, you realize your actions are excessive and unreasonable but you're unable to stop them. Compulsions include behaviors like checking several or even hundreds of times daily to make sure your stove is turned off or your doors are locked. Repeating a name, phrase, or action over and over also qualifies as a compulsion, as does taking an excessively slow and methodical approach to daily activities so that you spend hours organizing and arranging objects, or hoarding them. Hoarders are unable to throw away useless items, such as old newspapers, junk mail, even broken appliances. When hoarding reaches epic proportions, whole rooms can be filled with saved items.

OCD usually starts gradually, most often in adolescence or early adulthood. Unlike adults, children with OCD do not realize that their obsessions and compulsions are excessive.

To be diagnosed with this disorder, your obsessions and/or compulsions must take up at least one hour every day and interfere with normal routines (for example, if you can't make left turns when driving), occupational functioning, social activities, or relationships. You may feel the need to avoid certain situations. If you're obsessed with cleanliness, you may not be able to use public rest rooms.

Questions your physician may ask to determine whether you have OCD include . . .

1. Do you have unwanted ideas, images, or impulses that seem silly, nasty, or horrible?
2. Do you worry constantly about dirt, germs, or chemicals?
3. Are you excessively worried that something bad will happen if you forget something important, like turning off appliances or locking the door?
4. Do you keep many things you don't use because you can't throw them away?
5. Do you avoid situations or people you worry about hurting by angry words or actions?

Laura, age thirty-one, could not leave her house unless she washed her hands ten times. She'd taken biochemistry in college and knew humans swim in a sea of bacteria and viruses and she feared the dirt and disease-causing organisms in her environment. The hand-washing seemed to help at first, but then her skin became chapped and red, and she knew she had to stop it. But no matter how hard she tried, she couldn't stop washing. Her primary-care physician diagnosed her with obsessive-compulsive disorder and started her on a drug regimen.

■ Post-Traumatic Stress Disorder (PTSD)

Exposure to traumas, especially life-threatening ones, such as a serious accident, a natural disaster, war, or witnessing the death (or threat of death) of another person, or being assaulted can result in PTSD when the aftermath of the experience interferes with daily functioning. Common symptoms include avoiding activities, situations, people, and/or conversations associated with the event. Responses to trauma can include feelings of intense fear, helplessness, and/or horror, reexperiencing the event in thought or recurrent dreams, numbness and loss of interest in surroundings (detachment), inability to sleep, anxious feelings, being easily startled, irritability, angry outbursts, extreme vigilance, and a sense that your life opportunities have shrunk.

PTSD can occur at any age, although older adults rarely have it. Young children who have suffered a trauma may have nightmares, relive the event through play, and complain of headaches and stomachaches. Symptoms usually occur between three and six months after the trauma. In some cases, especially when the trauma is too terrible to allow into awareness, it could be years before symptoms appear. For these sufferers, symptoms are often triggered by the anniversary of the trauma or by the experience of another traumatic event.

For PTSD to be diagnosed, your symptoms must be present for more than a month and must result in decreased ability to work, socialize, and participate in other areas of daily functioning.

Your physician will probably ask you the following questions . . .

1. Have you experienced or witnessed a life-threatening event that caused intense fear, helplessness, or horror?
2. Do you reexperience the event and feel numb or detached, avoid thinking or talking about it, avoid activities or people who remind you of it, blank on important parts of it, lose interest in significant activities in your life, or sense your life will never be normal again?
3. Are you troubled by two or more of the following— problems sleeping, irritability or outbursts of anger, problems concentrating, feeling "on guard," or startling easily?

Jeff, age forty-one, came back from active duty in Iraq. Four of his buddies had died when their jeep passed over a land mine. He was thrown from the vehicle, but his buddies were killed. His physical injuries were severe enough for him to be sent back to the United States. In the VA hospital, Jeff lost interest in living and tried to hang himself. He began to have flashbacks of the incident in Iraq, couldn't keep his mind on a TV show, startled easily, couldn't sleep, and had unpredictable outbursts of anger. His nurse practitioner diagnosed him with post-traumatic stress disorder.

▌Social Phobia

If you have an intense fear and embarrassment in social or performance situations, you may be suffering from *social phobia*. If this is the case, you may be acutely aware of the physical signs of your anxiety (blushing, palpitations, tremors, sweating, diarrhea, confusion) and worry that others will notice, judge them, and think poorly of you. This kind of anxiety can lead to a panic attack when you are faced with a social situation or avoidance of the activity altogether.

If you suffer from social phobia, you tend to be sensitive to criticism and rejection, have difficulty asserting yourself, and suffer from low self-esteem. Common situations that bring out social phobia are performance related (speaking in public or to strangers, fear of meeting new people, writing, eating, and/or drinking in public).

Onset of social phobia is mid-to-late adolescence, but children may also exhibit symptoms. In childhood, the condition includes excessive shyness, clinging behavior, tantrums, mutism, decline in school performance, and avoidance of school and social activities with peers.

To diagnose social phobia, your physician may ask you . . .

1. Are you troubled by an intense and persistent fear of a social situation in which people might judge you?
2. Are you worried you might be humiliated by your actions?
3. Do you worry people will notice you are blushing, sweating, trembling, or showing other signs of anxiety?
4. Do you think your worry is excessive or unreasonable?
5. Do you go to great lengths to avoid participating in an uncomfortable situation?
6. In an uncomfortable social situation do you experience pounding heart, sweating, trembling or shaking, short-

ness of breath, choking, chest pain, nausea or abdominal discomfort, "jelly" legs, dizziness, feelings of unreality or being detached from yourself, fear of losing control or "going crazy," fear of dying, numbness or tingling sensations, chills or hot flashes?

7. Do any of these experiences interfere with your daily life?

■ Specific Phobia

Specific phobia refers to a discomfort, including a panic attack, due to an object or situation that interferes with daily routine, with employment (for example, missing out on a promotion because of a fear of flying), or with social life (for example, inability to go on a date to a crowded restaurant). If you have a phobia, you recognize that your reaction to the object or situation is unreasonable but are unable to control it. As a result, you may dread the object or situation, and try to avoid it.

Specific phobia may have its beginning in childhood, and is often brought on by a traumatic event, such as being bitten by a dog (leading to a dog phobia), almost being pushed off a high place (leading to fear of heights), and so forth. Fear of specific animals is the most common specific phobia. This condition can exist with panic disorder and agoraphobia.

Your physician may ask the following questions to diagnose your specific phobia . . .

1. Are you troubled by discomfort in social situations?
2. Are you fearful of places or situations where getting help or escape might be difficult, such as in a crowd, on a bridge, or alone in a high place?
3. Do you experience shortness of breath or a racing heart for no apparent reason?

4. Do you suffer from a persistent and unreasonable discomfort when flying, in a high place, around animals, or at the sight of blood or other objects or situations?
5. Are you unable to travel without a companion?

Robby, age thirty-five, suffered from a fear of being bitten by a large dog. As a youngster, he had witnessed his brother being bitten by a rabid rottweiler. As Robby got older, he almost forgot about his fear until a neighbor bought a large dog that barked at him one day when he was out for a walk. Robby started to sweat and feel dizzy. His heart raced and he couldn't catch his breath. After that, he stopped taking walks and consulted his physician. Robby was diagnosed with specific phobia.

■ Other Diagnostic Questions

It's not unusual to have depression or substance abuse while suffering from an anxiety disorder. So, in addition to the questions listed above for each condition, your physician might also ask you . . .

1. More days than not, do you feel sad or depressed, uninterested in life, or worthless or guilty?
2. During the last year has the use of alcohol or drugs placed you in a dangerous situation, gotten you arrested, resulted in your failure to fulfill important responsibilities (work, school, or family), or continued despite causing problems for you and/or your loved ones?

■ Your Anxiety Condition

Go back and see which of the anxiety conditions described in this chapter is most bothersome to you. As you work through this book, pay special attention to the symptoms you have and think about medical and self-actions that may be beneficial. The next chapter describes the effects prescribed medications may have on you.

4

Anxiety, Your Brain, and Medication

More than 100,000 chemical reactions occur in your brain every second. This amazing organ is capable of more than anyone can yet imagine, but when anxiety rises, it can interfere with normal brain functioning.

■ Your Brain and Emotions

Three parts of your brain are especially important to your anxiety. Your *hypothalamus,* a pea-sized structure in your brain's central core, controls biological rhythms that influence sleep cycles, energy levels, pleasure, and other important emotional experiences. When your hypothalamus isn't functioning properly, you may feel fatigued, yet still have problems sleeping.

Your *limbic system,* which surrounds the hypothalamus, is often called the "emotional brain." It's a launching pad for felt emotions. When you feel afraid or anxious, the experience is set in motion by chemical activity taking place in the limbic system. This set of structures also inhibits and controls emotional actions.

The *prefrontal cortex,* the front part of your brain, inhibits emotional reactions, maintains attention and concentration, and assists in complex thinking and problem solving. Your brain has many interconnections between the frontal lobes and the limbic system. Although there is convincing evidence that the frontal cortex is dysfunctional in some psychiatric disorders, there is little or no proof of actual tissue damage.

Normal functioning of your brain is dependent on the appropriate action of *neurons* (nerve cells) responsible for turning particular brain centers on and off, somewhat like turning a TV or computer on and off. The neurotransmitting chemicals released by particular nerve cells are given the name of that cell. Thus, a *dopamine nerve cell* is a cell that manufactures and releases dopamine, while the nerve cells that release serotonin are called *serotonin nerve cells*, and so on. The list of nerve cells, neurotransmitters, and amino acids implicated in affecting mood and behavior is growing and includes: serotonin, dopamine, norepinephrine, gamma-amino butyric acid (GABA), glycine, histamine, acetylcholine, glutamate, and aspartate. (See chapter 5 for more information on how the food you eat can help you to develop healthy neurotransmitters.)

One of your brain's many jobs is to produce chemicals that help you remember, go to sleep, think clearly, and feel good. *Endorphins* are your brain's painkiller, and they are three times more potent than morphine.

Another opiate-like chemical in your brain and spinal cord is *serotonin*, a hormone. When your serotonin level is low, depression usually follows. When your brain produces serotonin, tension and anxiety are eased. When your brain produces dopamine or norepinephrine, you are more alert and react more quickly.

It is theorized that a dysfunction in just a tiny percentage of total brain cells can lead to a psychiatric disorder. What has not been proved is whether these chemical changes are responsible for causing the psychiatric disorder. Some experts, including Breggin and

Cohen, believe psychiatric drugs can cause brain-chemistry imbalances and set off subsequent attempts by the brain to compensate that can create lifelong damage.

▋ Drugs and Your Brain

Psychiatric drugs became part of the top moneymakers for the pharmaceutical industry in the mid-1970s. By then, drugs to treat anxiety and depression had been developed. Since then, their use has skyrocketed. According to the new president of the American Psychiatric Association, "Psychiatry's relationship with drug companies is rife with the appearance of conflict of interest and frankly with conflict of interest itself."

Breggin and Cohen maintain that some anti-anxiety drugs, such as Prozac, Ritalin, and Xanax, actually *cause* a chemical imbalance, rather than correct it. Peter R. Breggin, M.D., an expert in psychiatric drugs and their negative effects, says that all the commonly used minor tranquilizers, with the possible exception of BuSpar, are sedatives, or central-nervous-system depressants, and create clinical effects similar to alcohol and barbiturates. Bear in mind that one of the most common side effects of sedatives is depression!

All minor tranquilizers impair physical coordination and mental alertness, which is why it's dangerous to drive or use other mechanical devices when taking them. Even at low doses these drugs can impact your brain waves on routine EEGs, especially in the frontal lobe of the brain.

Most drugs interact with specific receptors in your brain to produce their effects. *Receptors* are structures located on the outside surface of nerve cells. These structures interact with a variety of chemicals, including medications. Think of a chemical as a key and the receptor as a lock. But it's not quite that simple. Other substances, including hormones, can also bind to these receptors and interact with them in certain psychiatric conditions, according to Stephen M. Stahl, MD, PhD.

According to Samuel H. Barondes, all psychiatric medications work on the same neurotransmitters—primarily dopamine, serotonin, norepinephrine, and gamma-aminobutyric acid (GABA). Although drug companies would like us to believe psychiatric disorders are the result of an excess or deficiency of these chemicals that can be fixed by taking a medication, the researchers who know how drugs work and how they effect the brain still don't know how they effect the cause of an anxiety disorder, if in fact they do. Moreover, many psychiatric drugs frequently bind to more than one receptor, and so have more than one effect. Some of these effects can be worse than anxiety.

Medications are not magic bullets. They do not target a receptor upon entering your body, appear magically at their goal, perform their work, and then disappear. This false notion completely ignores the facts. It is possible that you can take anti-anxiety drugs, feel better, and experience no short-term side effects. Be aware that these drugs have not been tested for long-term use or on the unique individual that is you. (Research results only present averages, not individual responses.)

▌Be Cautious When Taking Anti-Anxiety Drugs

There are at least three reasons to be cautious when taking anti-anxiety drugs:

1. drugs can cause damage as they go through your body
2. drugs don't necessarily stop having effects as soon as they have done the work they were intended to do
3. many anti-anxiety drugs are addictive and can create severe withdrawal symptoms.

This is a caution against using any medication injudiciously. Work with your health care practitioner to monitor drug use carefully so you can decide when the costs are outweighing the benefits, and stop using any medication once it's no longer needed or if it creates dangerous side effects. You may have to remind your health care practitioner how long you've been on a drug, and inquire whether a liver function test or some other test is needed.

Keep in mind that quick and easy treatments for difficult problems are rare, if not nonexistent. Still, your hope for a miracle drug may be strong, especially these days when the drug industry spends more than twice as much on marketing and administration as it does on drug research and development. It's nearly impossible to turn on a TV without seeing an ad for this or that drug. The side effects are glossed over and many are promoted for uses that have never even been researched.

Keeping this in mind, you might want to consider becoming one of the many individuals who refuses to take prescription drugs, and thereby avoid their irritating and sometimes dangerous side effects. This book can help you do just that by showing you how to change your eating patterns, participate in daily vigorous exercise, use deep relaxation or meditation, alter your self-talk and basic beliefs, and find a life purpose. If you are so debilitated by anxiety that it's impossible for you to leave your home, you can work with a cognitive-behavioral nurse-therapist who can use anxiety-reduction techniques to enable you to function. (See chapter 9.)

Keep several things in mind when considering whether to take drugs to quell your anxiety. Remember that *drugs don't cure you*. They only work on symptoms. That is, they may (or may not) reduce your anxiety, but they work only as long as you take the drug, and will do nothing to stop the real cause of your anxiety. This means they provide temporary relief, while only nonchemical lifestyle changes can produce complete and enduring relief.

Another important fact to keep in mind is that *all drugs have side effects*. Drugs are prescribed for one of their many effects, but to get that result, you may have to put up with a variety of side effects. In fact, many individuals stop taking their prescribed anti-anxiety drugs because of their annoying side effects.

Also remember that *any drug that is strong enough to have a significant effect has the potential for rebound and withdrawal symptoms*. Breggin and Cohen point out that drugs that suppress anxiety or induce sleep when used over the long term should always be suspected of causing irreversible mental dysfunction.

You can also develop a reliance on drugs, so if you're not currently taking them, I hope you will give the methods in this book a fair trial before electing to take them.

If you're already taking a drug and decide to stop, only do so in concert with your health-care practitioner. Together you can find the best way to end your dependence so that you don't have a very negative reaction. Gradually tapering off is the only safe way to stop taking a drug. This gradual approach is especially important if you're taking a tranquilizer, because going cold turkey can be dangerous.

If you do decide to take medications, always be informed about what you're taking, the correct dosage, what effects to expect, and any dangerous side effects and what to do about them if they occur. This holds true for all drugs, not just medications prescribed to reduce anxiety. (For example, one study has linked oral contraceptives to panic disorder. Once women taking triphasal oral contraceptive stopped taking it, their panic attacks disappeared. Researchers concluded that the oral contraceptives precipitated panic disorder with agoraphobia.)

■ Types of Anti-Anxiety Drugs

Several kinds of medications are prescribed for high anxiety. The major ones are tranquilizers, antidepressants, and non-benzodiazepines.

Benzodiazepine Tranquilizers

The minor tranquilizers, or *benzodiazepines*, include Ativan (lorazepam), Centrax (prazepam), Klonopin (clonazepam), Xanax (alprazolam), Serum (oxazepam), and Tranxene (chlorazepate). Benzodiazepine sedatives used for sleep include Dalmane (flurazepam), Halcion (triazolam), Versed (midazolam), and Restoril (temazepam).

These drugs reduce anxiety by depressing the activity of your central nervous system. All these drugs have the serious side effect of making you physically dependent on them, which means you'll have a difficult time when you try to stop taking them, especially if you take high doses over a long period of time. If you're taking Xanax or Halcion, withdrawal symptoms can occur daily between doses, worsening the original anxiety symptoms. To top it off, in one clinical trial, 70 percent of persons taking Halcion "developed memory loss, depression and paranoia." Breggin and Cohen state that, like most psychiatric drugs, Halcion eventually causes an increase of the very symptoms that the drug is supposed to ameliorate.

Besides addiction and withdrawal reactions, if you take these drugs, you can face problems similar to those experienced by people who abuse alcohol, including intoxication without realizing it, slowed thinking, slurred speech, lack of coordination, clumsiness, impaired walking, tremor, poor judgment, drowsiness, drugged feelings, and hangovers with amnesia. These drugs work by impairing brain function and pose a risk of irreversible mental dysfunction. Students taking these drugs can experience severe amnesia and forget the material they studied.

These drugs may cause drowsiness, so avoid driving or other tasks that require alertness. Other possible side effects include depression, apathy, fatigue, decreased activity, light-headedness, memory impairment, disorientation, amnesia, restlessness, confusion, crying, delirium, headaches, slurred speech, loss of voice, stupor, seizures, coma, fainting, rigidity, tremor, abnormal muscle tone, vertigo, dizziness, euphoria, nervousness, irritability, difficulty concentrating, agitation, inability to perform complex mental functions, paralysis of half the body, unsteadiness, loss of coordination, strange dreams, glassy-eyed appearance, increased anxiety or hyperactivity, behavior problems, hysteria, psychosis, suicidal tendencies, constipation, diarrhea, dry mouth, coated tongue, sore gums, nausea, changes in appetite, vomiting, difficulty swallowing, increased salivation, stomach inflammation, incontinence, changes in sex drive, urinary and menstrual problems, changes in heart rhythm and blood pressure, cardiovascular collapse, retention of fluid in the face and ankles, palpitations, visual disturbances, twitching of the eyeballs, decreased hearing, nasal congestion, auditory disturbances, rashes, itching, hair loss or growth, hiccups, fever, sweating, tingling in the extremities, muscular disturbances, growth of breasts in males, milk production in the breasts of females, breathing difficulties, hepatitis or jaundice, changes in blood-cell counts, decrease in body weight, swelling of lymph nodes, and joint pain.

These drugs may increase levels or prolong the effects of barbiturates, narcotics, phenytoin, probenecid, and sedating antihistamines. They have potentially dangerous interactions with digoxin. When combined with alcohol and other medications, Xanax can cause death, even in low doses. When taking this medication or any other, never take more than is prescribed, and always ask to take the lowest dose that achieves the prescribed effect.

Xanax is the most popular tranquilizer and is used most often to treat anxiety disorders. If you have nonspecific, generalized anxiety, Xanax will probably be prescribed for you in doses of 0.5–2 mg/day. If you have panic attacks, your health-care practitioner may prescribe 2–9 mg/day. Xanax is sometimes used temporarily for acute anxiety or agoraphobia.

Xanax, and other anti-anxiety drugs, are central nervous system (CNS) depressants. They affect the neurotransmitter gamma-aminobutyric acid (GABA) that facilitates communication between brain cells. Because brain cell activity is slowed, they can produce a drowsy or calming effect on those suffering from anxiety. In high doses, CNS depressants can be used as general anesthetics.

At first, Xanax may seem beneficial, but as your body becomes accustomed to the effects of the drug, its calming effects disappear as you develop a tolerance to it. This is when the potential for abuse of the drug occurs, as larger doses are needed to achieve the same initial effects.

While small doses may relieve tension, large doses produce staggering, blurred vision, impaired thinking, slurred speech, impaired perception of time and space, slowed reflexes and reduced sensitivity to pain. Accidental overdoses occur when children swallow pills—always keep all medication out of reach of children or adolescents—or when adults with increased tolerance are unsure of how many to take.

Researchers studying the 24 medical examiners in Florida in 2000 and 2001 concluded that in 939 cases of death (a tripling from 284 cases in 2000), prescription painkillers and benzodiazepine drugs such as Xanax or Valium were found. A U.S. Department of Justice website (www.usdoj.gov/ndic/pubs07/717.odd.htm) reported that the number of admissions to South Carolina publicly funded treatment centers for benzodiazepine abuse more than doubled from FY 1998 (43) to FY 2000 (99).

As a parent or individual, if you suspect you or someone else in the family is abusing Xanax, you can get a definitive answer by using a simple, private urine drug-testing kit available at www.home drugtestingkit.com/zshop.

When prescribed an anti-anxiety drug, always read all the information provided by the pharmacist and beware of potential interactions with other drugs, foods, and substances such as alcohol.

A major problem with Xanax and other benzodiazepines is that they blunt not only your anxiety but your other feelings as well. I've had clients tell me that tranquilizers are like mental straitjackets that make them feel less human. If you're simultaneously trying to work out your feelings in psychotherapy, tranquilizers will interfere with this process, especially if you're on high doses of the drug. Like many other drugs, Xanax will only take away your anxiety, but it won't remove the source of your feelings. When taking only tranquilizers, and not examining your lifestyle you may never be able to find out what is causing your anxiety or learn how to prevent or control your reactions.

A few people report becoming more emotional, more hostile, and have difficulty sleeping when taking Xanax. Panic can be doubled and seizures can occur if the dose is reduced too rapidly or if Xanax is abruptly stopped once dependence develops.

Xanax interacts negatively with melatonin, kava, valerian, grapefruit juice, and many other drugs, foods, and herbs. If you have alcoholic liver disease, are obese, or have reduced liver or kidney function, dangerous levels of Xanax may accumulate in your body. If you decide to take Xanax, use it for a short period of time on as "as-needed" basis rather than daily over a long time. Because rapid withdrawal may be life threatening, tapering off the drug should be done only under medical supervision.

Halcion can cause depression and paranoia. It has been banned in England.

Versed can cause behavioral abnormalities, and its emotionally disturbing effects are long-lasting. According to Breggin and Cohen, Versed should be considered a very hazardous drug.

Withdrawal from Klonopin may be easy for some people, although I've had clients who were unable to get off the drug completely even after protracted withdrawal. Abrupt withdrawal from these drugs is dangerous and can produce panic attacks, severe anxiety, confusion, muscle tension, irritability, insomnia, paranoid delusions, hallucinations, memory impairment, vomiting, headache, loss of appetite, tremor, voice changes, and even seizures.

In sum, Xanax and the other minor tranquilizers are more help-ful for acute anxiety on a short-term basis than for long-lasting con-ditions such as agoraphobia. If you do take these drugs for more than two years, and especially if you're over age fifty, you should have an evaluation of your liver function every six months or so.

Margaret, age thirty-three, a computer programmer, suffered from severe anxiety and panic attacks. Her physician prescribed Xanax, at a dosage of 5 mg a day. When Margaret started to develop fre-quent headaches, loss of appetite, strange dreams, and thoughts about killing herself, she increased her dosage without telling her physician. Luckily, her sister walked in when Margaret was trying to cut her wrists and brought her to the hospital. During her stay, her medications were reevaluated and she was taken off Xanax. She joined a cognitive-behavioral therapy group and learned ways to control her anxiety.

Antidepressants

Antidepressant medications are often prescribed to treat panic at-tacks, or agoraphobia with panic attacks. There are four different types of antidepressants:

1. *Cyclic antidepressants* such as Elavil (amitriptyline), Tofranil (imipramine), Pamelor (nortriptyline), Surmontil (trimipramine), Desyrel (trazodone), Sinequan (doxepin), Norpramin (desipramine), Vivactil (protriptyline), and Anafranil (clomipramine). According to Mindell and Hopkins, potential side effects or adverse reactions in-clude dry mouth, blurred vision, problems focusing, increased eye pressure that can lead to glaucoma, dilation of the pupils, constipa-tion, dysfunction of parts of the small intestine, urinary problems, drastic dips in blood pressure when going from lying to sitting or from sitting to standing, high blood pressure, heart rhythm abnor-malities, congestive heart failure, stroke, electrocardiogram changes

(suggesting damage to heart tissue), confusion, disturbed concentration, hallucinations, disorientation, impaired memory, feelings of unreality, delusions, anxiety, nervousness, restlessness, agitation, panic, insomnia, nightmares, mania, worsening of psychotic symptoms, drowsiness, dizziness, weakness, fatigue, headache, depression, excessive tension in the muscles or artery walls, sleep disorders, psychosomatic disorders, yawning, abnormal dreaming, migraines, depersonalization, irritability and mood swings, numbness, tingling, hyperactivity, lack of coordination, tremors, peripheral neuropathy (nerve changes in legs and arms), seizures, twitching, partial paralysis, allergic reactions (rash, itching, swelling), changes in blood-cell counts, nausea, vomiting, loss of appetite, diarrhea, flatulence, trouble swallowing, strange taste in the mouth, increased salivation, abdominal cramps, inflammation (stomach, throat, or esophagus), black tongue, indigestion, breast development and testicular swelling (in men), breast enlargement, spontaneous flow of milk, vaginitis and menstrual difficulties, changes in sex drive, painful ejaculation, voiding of urine during the night, cystitis, urinary-tract infection, changes in blood glucose levels, increase secretion of hormones (prolactin and vasopressin, an antidiuretic), pharnygitis, laryngitis, sinusitis, coughing, spasm of the breathing airways, nosebleed, shortness of breath, problems speaking, ringing of the ears, excessive tearing of the eyes, conjunctivitis, difference in the size of the pupils, inner-ear inflammation, eye allergy symptoms, nasal congestion, excessive appetite, body-weight changes, increased sweating, high body temperature, flushing, chills, hair loss, dental problems, abnormal skin odor, chest pain, fever, bad breath, thirst, back pain and joint aches, and increased sensitivity to the sun.

Henry, age twenty-two, a college senior, suffered from panic attacks. His primary-care physician prescribed Elavil. After two months Henry began to experience confusion, disturbed concentration, extreme anxiety, and worry that someone was trying to break into his room and poison him. His roommate took him to the university hospital ER, where he was admitted to the psychiatric unit and diagnosed with schizophrenia. When Henry was taken off Elavil his symptoms disappeared and he was discharged from the hospital. He worked with a cognitive-behavioral therapist on an outpatient basis and learned how to stay calm during stressful school situations.

2. MAO-inhibitors include Nardil (phenelzine), Parnate (tranyl-cypromine), and Marplan (isocarboxazid).These drugs can cause serious or even fatal rises in blood pressure when combined with: (1) foods that contain the amino acid tyramine, such as wine and certain meat; (2) stimulants and antidepressants; (3) over-the-counter medications, such as decongestants. If you are taking an MAO-inhibitor, you should be under close supervision by your physician. Be sure to watch for low blood pressure, extreme fevers, sexual dysfunction, daytime sleepiness, nighttime insomnia, muscle pain, and muscle spasms.

3. Selective serotonin reuptake inhibitors (SSRIs) include Prozac (fluoxetine), Zoloft (sertraline), and Paxil (paroxetine). These drugs are used primarily to treat panic disorder, agoraphobia (six to twelve months), and obsessive-compulsive disorder (long-term maintenance). The SSRIs may also be used for generalized anxiety, especially when combined with depression.

According to Mindell and Hopkins, potential side effects include nervousness, insomnia, drowsiness, fatigue, weakness, tremor, increased sweating, dizziness, anxiety (especially with Prozac), headache (especially with Paxil), dry mouth (with Zoloft and Paxil), male sexual dysfunction (Zoloft), altered appetite and weight, and constipation (Paxil), and loss of appetite, nausea, diarrhea, and stomach discomfort (Prozac and Zoloft). Although weight loss may occur at first, many individuals experience weight gain after a period of months, which may lead to obesity.

Over 40,000 reports of adverse effects from Prozac have been submitted to the Food and Drug Administration since it was first marketed. No other drug comes close, according to Breggin and Cohen. They also state that these drugs can produce effects similar to amphetamine or methamphetamine, including an artificial feeling of well-being or energy, anxiety, agitation, and insomnia. Effexor (see below) and Prozac are stimulating, while the others cause drowsiness or insomnia. Like the amphetamines, these drugs can cause manic psychoses, and can also lead to less caring and loving attention to family members, as well as sexual dysfunction with mates.

Withdrawal from the drug can lead to "crashing" into depression and suicidal thoughts and actions. Breggin and Cohen report seeing patients who became very disturbed and violent when dosage was reduced, and others who reported feeling tortured from within, which may be related to the drug's ability to cause self-destructive or violent behavior.

Numerous suicide and homicide cases have involved individuals who took SSRIs for as little as a few days. Because the drugs can cause agitation and anxiety, they may lead to increased use of alcohol and other calming drugs. SSRIs can cause drowsiness or dizziness. Use caution when driving, performing tasks requiring alertness, or operating machinery.

In research studies, between 15 and 21 percent of those on SSRIs stopped taking them due to unpleasant side effects. Rash, fever, joint pain, abnormal changes in blood-cell counts, swelling, excessive excretion of protein in the urine (indicating liver or kidney damage), and elevated enzymes in the bloodstream (also indicating tissue damage) have occurred in some people taking Prozac. If you are prescribed this drug and experience any of these symptoms, you are probably sensitive to it and should contact your health-care practitioner immediately to stop taking it. If you don't, you may end up having a life-threatening anaphylactic shock reaction. In these cases the life-threatening nature of the reaction trumps the potential "crashing" reaction.

> Connie, a thirty-eight-year-old university professor, was prescribed Prozac for her anxiety about lecturing to large groups of students. When she went to have her annual physical, the lab tests came back positive for liver and kidney damage. Her doctor immediately took her off Prozac and told her never to take the drug again because she was probably sensitive to it.

Serotonin syndrome is caused by taking an overdose of SSRIs or by an interaction of SSRIs with other drugs. It can be fatal. Symptoms include hallucinations, confusion, agitation, fever, fluctuating blood pressure, stiffness, irregular heartbeats, and seizures.

The effects of withdrawal from these drugs can include dizziness, headaches, nausea, poor concentration, fatigue, moodiness, and mental fogginess. Allow at least two weeks to slowly withdraw from these drugs and do it under the supervision of a health-care professional familiar with their use.

Clinical trials of these drugs have only lasted for five to sixteen weeks, except in the case of Prozac, which has been tested for up to a year. In other words, the long-term effects of these drugs have not been studied in any systematic fashion.

Avoid these drugs if you have impaired liver function, tend to be manic, have a history of seizures, or are using diuretics. If you are diabetic, Prozac can affect insulin levels, and your drug dose may need to be readjusted.

4. *Other Antidepressants* include Wellbutrin (bupropion), Asendin (amoxapine), Ludiomil (maprotiline), Remeron (mirtazapine), Effexor (venlafaxine), Serzone (nefazodone), and Desyrel (tra-zodone), and Zyban (buproprion).

Wellbutrin may be difficult to tolerate since its side effects in-clude anxiety and insomnia, and it can produce a high rate of seizures and cause anxiety, nightmares, and manic psychoses. Asendin is converted into a neuroleptic within the body. Neurolep-tics are chemical lobotomies that blunt the highest functions of the brain and result in apathy, indifference, emotional blandness, con-formity, and submissiveness, as well as reduction in all verbaliza-tions, including complaints or protests. According to Breggin and Cohen, these drugs are used in veterinary medicine to control vio-lent animals, but only for a short period of time because they are considered so dangerous.

Ludiomil may produce seizures and involuntary abnormal move-ments, and Remeron can induce sedation, dizziness, weight gain, and low blood pressure. Heart and blood vessel problems have been reported in connection with both drugs, as well as toxic psychoses, including mania and delirium.

Effexor's potentially negative effects are similar to Prozac's and include anxiety, nervousness, insomnia, loss of appetite, and weight loss. Other effects of Effexor include agitation, mania, hostility, paranoid reactions, psychotic depression, toxic psychosis, and high blood pressure. Serzone is more likely to cause sleepiness than in-somnia and can produce light-headedness, confusion, memory im-pairment, and low blood pressure, as well as hostility, paranoid reactions, suicidal thoughts and suicide attempts, depersonalization, and hallucinations. Desyrel is apt to cause sedation, dizziness, and fainting, as well as heart problems if you already have a cardiac di-agnosis, and a kind of irreversible penile erection that may require surgical correction.

Drawbacks of all antidepressants include bothersome side effects (at least for the first week or two), which can be reduced by starting off with a very low dosage and gradually increasing the amount over two or three weeks. Other drawbacks are that antidepressants take two to four weeks to take effect, and panic and depressive symptoms can return after withdrawing from them.

Non-Benzodiazepines

Found in this category are Ambien (zolpidem), Atarax or Vistaril (hydroxyzine), Amytal (amobarbital), Butisol (butabarbital), Mebaral (Mephobarbital), Nembutal (pentobarbital), phenobarbital (generic), Seconal (secobarbital), and beta-adrenergic blockers (or, beta blockers), including Inderal (propranolol) and Tenormin (atenolol), BuSpar (buspirone), Miltown (meprobamate), and Trancopel (chlormezanone). Ambien, a sleep aid, can cause drowsiness, confusion, awkward gait, headache, nausea, fatigue (including dizziness and lack of coordination leading to falls), psychosis, hallucinations, nightmares, sensory disturbances, memory problems, and bizarre or dangerous behavior.

Atarax and Vistaril have antihistamine and sedative qualities.

Barbiturates (Amytal, Butisol, Mebaral, Nembutal, phenobarbital and Seconal) are prescribed to induce sleep and reduce anxiety. They are highly addictive and can produce toxic symptoms comparable to alcohol, including sedation, dizziness or light-headedness, vomiting, diarrhea, muscle cramps, slurred speech, poor judgment, clumsiness, and hangovers. They can also produce the opposite of what is wanted, namely hallucination, depression, excitement, hyperactivity, and aggression. Research has shown that phenobarbital can reduce IQ measurably.

Audrey, nineteen, a college student, went to the college health service because she was so anxious about taking tests and feared she wasn't going to be able to stay in school. Seconal was prescribed to help her sleep and reduce her anxiety. Three days later, the college police picked her up on the road for acting confused, having slurred speech, and being unable to walk in a straight line. Her roommate, who was a student nurse, took her to see the physician who had prescribed the medication. Audrey was taken off Seconal and referred to an advanced psychiatric nurse practitioner to learn anxiety-reducing measures, which she did. A week later, Audrey was able to return to classes.

Beta blockers block muscular manifestations of anxiety, but may not reduce the internal experience of anxiety. They may be given in a single dose to relieve severe physical symptoms before a high-performance situation, such as public speaking, a job interview, final examinations, or a musical recital. The downside of these drugs is that they can cause congestive heart failure, heart attacks, strokes and asthma, irregular heartbeats, and may worsen blood vessel problems, which reduce circulation to the extremities, such as in diabetes. If you have asthma, avoid these drugs because they may trigger life-threatening airway spasms.

It's not known how BuSpar (buspirone) works, but it is prescribed for the treatment of anxiety. Possible side effects include temporary or permanent damage to the nervous system, drug dependence, sedation, and withdrawal reactions. Adverse reactions have included dizziness, drowsiness, restlessness, nervousness, insomnia, nausea, light-headedness, headaches, numbness, dream disturbances, fatigue, sore throat, tinnitus (ringing in ears), and nasal congestion. Mindell and Hopkins advise thinking twice before taking this drug as there are so many other safer alternatives.

Buspirone may raise levels or prolong the effects of Haloperidol and MAO-inhibitors. An ordinary starting dose is 5 mg two to three times a day. It takes from two to three weeks before the effect of this medication is achieved. Some individuals get more anxious than they were prior to taking the drug.

Miltown is addictive and subject to abuse and can cause many of the adverse effects evoked by the other sedative drugs. Trancopel can also provoke many adverse effects, including depression, confusion, and severe skin rashes.

■ Procedure for Weaning Yourself from a Drug

If you've decided that you want to stop relying on prescription medications, observe the following guidelines:

1. Gain a level of mastery of the basic strategies for overcoming anxiety and panic presented in this book. For starters, establish a daily practice of deep relaxation and exercise, along with skills in deep abdominal breathing, self-talk, and muscle relaxation. Make sure you have adopted a healthier eating program and explore the use of herbs. These skills will help you through the withdrawal period from a drug. Be assured that any resurgence of anxiety is temporary and shouldn't persist once you've completed the withdrawal process.

2. Consult with your physician to set up a program to gradually taper off the dosage of your medication. The tapering-off period is dependent on the dose you're taking, but may go on for up to two months or longer.

3. Be prepared to increase your reliance on your new skills learned from working with this book during the tapering-off period. Additional skills you will need during this period include identifying and expressing your feelings and coping skills. Using these skills will provide you with the self-confidence to master your anxiety and panic without relying on medication.

▮ Working with Your Physician

Before taking any medication, make sure you are fully aware of all the potential side effects and limitations of any drug you are prescribed. It is your physician's responsibility to (1) obtain a complete history of your symptoms, (2) inform you of your diagnosis as well as the possible side effects and limitations for any drug you are asked to take, and (3) obtain your written informed consent to try out a medication.

As added protection, look up the prescription of a medication you're considering in the *Physicians' Desk Reference* (PDR). Your physician probably has a copy in the office, or you can look up the drug in the reference section of your library or search for the particular drug online.

Your responsibility is to fully inform your physician about any other drugs or supplements you are currently taking. Withholding information could lead to being prescribed a drug that interacts in a dangerous way with what you are already taking. It's also important to tell your physician about any allergic reactions to drugs you've had, if you are pregnant, and if you are taking any over-the-counter medications or herbs.

Once you've exchanged this important information both of you will be fully informed, and you can make a mutual decision about whether taking a particular medication is in your best interest. If your current physician is unwilling to take this kind of collaborative approach, I strongly urge you to find another doctor—one who will. (See chapter 12 for more information.)

While anti-anxiety drugs may work well for you, use them safely by

- always asking to take the smallest dose that achieves the prescribed effect

- never taking more than is prescribed
- asking for drug literature from your pharmacist and reading and heeding it
- reevaluating their use periodically by asking your health-care practitioner for a liver function or other type of test to determine negative side effects when you've been on the drug for more than six months
- never changing dosages or stopping a drug without gradually weaning yourself off it; always work even more closely with your health-care practitioner in this case.

PART TWO

Holistic Approaches to Anxiety

5

Nutrition

What you eat has a direct effect on your body's chemistry. It's been known for decades that food affects mood. Certain foods and substances you ingest can create stress and anxiety, while others calm you down. You may not recognize how what you eat affects you, but there is a simple way to tune into these interactions.

> Henny, a forty-year-old nurse, experienced high anxiety and panic attacks when she had to go above the second floor in a building. She also complained of insomnia and heart palpitations. When we examined her eating habits, I pointed out that drinking coffee and eating sugary foods was probably contributing to her anxiety. When she changed her eating patterns, her anxiety lessened.

Keep a Food/Mood Diary for several weeks and you'll begin to identify the connection between what you eat and how you feel. Here is a sample of Henny's food/mood diary:

Date/Time	Food/Drink	Mental State	Physical State	Unusual Behaviors
Tues. 1:00 P.M.	cup of coffee & doughnut	drowsy	fatigued	
2:00 P.M.	cup of coffee	jittery, anxious		
4:00 P.M.	candy bar & Coke			
4:20 P.M.		panic attack		

▌ Substances That Aggravate Anxiety

Caffeine

Several of my clients could directly trace their sleeping problems and sometimes their first panic attack to caffeine. Coffee is the most obvious, but there are many other sources of caffeine, including tea, cocoa, Coca-Cola, Dr. Pepper, Mountain Dew, Tab, Pepsi, chocolate, and even decaffeinated coffee! Many over-the-counter drugs also contain caffeine, among them Anacin, Caffedrine, Empirin, Excedrin, Pre-mens Forte, Vanquish, Vivarin, and No-Doz.

Caffeine stimulates several different parts of your body. It releases adrenaline into your body just as if you're undergoing stress. It also pours norepinephrine into your brain, causing you to feel more awake and alert. By keeping you in a constant state of arousal, your adrenal glands and other portions of your body are kept in a state of emergency. This can be very stressful. This kind of over-arousal makes you more vulnerable to anxiety and panic. Add to that stress the fact that caffeine acts as a diuretic that pushes calming minerals and antistress B vitamins out in your urine. Caffeine is not something you want to subject your body to.

Wean yourself off caffeine, but do it slowly. Gradually mix in a half cup of decaffeinated with half a cup of coffee. Slowly increase the decaffeinated coffee over a week or so until you are drinking de-caffeinated coffee only. Better yet, do the same with caffeinated tea and herbal tea. Do the same with cocoa and carob and chocolate candy and carob candy. Also, start drinking noncaffeinated sodas or mixing them as suggested above.

Salt

Salt, especially table salt, stresses your body and can deplete it of potassium (an important mineral that keeps your nervous system healthy) and raise blood pressure, putting an extra strain on your heart. In one study, students with higher levels of anxiety reported higher salt consumption and lower levels of exercise. Avoid salting your food and use a natural salt substitute such as tamari, or use herbs such as basil and oregano or lemon to spice your food. Avoid buying canned or frozen foods that list salt as an ingredient.

Saturated Fats

Foods high in saturated fats such as fried foods, hamburgers, and french fries, lead to sluggishness and fatigue. Fats inhibit the synthesis of neurotransmitters and cause blood cells to become sticky and clump together, resulting in poor brain circulation.

Sugar

Americans, on average, eat sixty-five pounds of sugar a year, way too much of the simple sugars that can create anxiety and panic. What your brain needs is naturally occurring sugar (glucose) to function by burning it for fuel. Much of this form of sugar is de-rived from carbohydrate foods such as cereal, bread, potatoes, veg-etables, fruits (especially grapefruit and apples), pasta, and brown rice. Simple sugars from cakes, pies, candy, and other sweets are problematic for your body because they tend to break down too quickly, stressing your body by causing an oversecretion of in-sulin from your pancreas, and resulting in an imbalance in sugar metabolism. At this point your blood sugar level sinks so low you feel twitchy, light-headed, and anxious. Once blood sugar is so low, your adrenal glands kick in and "help" with an injection of cortisol, which can make you feel panicky, ready to "fight or flee."

Excessive sugar intake can also result in withdrawal symptoms. Symptoms of these imbalances include anxiety, trembling, weakness or unsteadiness, light-headedness, irritability, and palpitations. These are the exact symptoms of a panic attack. To eliminate these symptoms, modify your eating patterns by

1. Substituting fruits (other than dried fruits) for sugar.
2. Avoiding fruit juices or diluting them 1:1 with water.
3. Eliminating simple sugars from your diet. These include candy, ice cream, frozen yogurt and some regular yogurt (read the label), desserts, Coke and Pepsi and other sodas containing sugar; corn syrup, corn sweeteners, fructose, and honey.
4. Reducing or eliminating simple starches from your diet. Replace them with complex carbohydrates that take longer to digest, including whole-grain breads and cereals, and vegetables.
5. Having a complex carbohydrate or protein snack halfway between meals, such as a slice of cheese on a whole-grain cracker, a handful of nuts, peanut butter on a banana or apple. A turkey sandwich on whole-grain bread is a good combination if you want to raise your levels of "feel good" serotonin. The turkey can also help you sleep. Eating five or six small meals a day will also keep you balanced and less anxious because it helps you maintain a stable blood sugar.

■ Missing Nutrients That Can Lead to Anxiety

You can experience anxiety if your body is missing important nutrients. This section discusses the more important ones.

Minerals

Minerals work in concert and need to be available at the same time for best results. *Calcium* is a natural tranquilizer and *magnesium* helps to relieve anxiety, tension, nervousness, muscle spasms, and tics. When calcium is present in insufficient amounts in your body, you can experience heart palpitations, insomnia, muscle cramps, nervousness, numbness, delusions, and hyperactivity. When you don't get enough magnesium, you can feel nervous and weak, have insomnia, be irritable, or have a rapid heartbeat. Twitching can also result, as can an imbalance in your acid-alkali balance. When experiencing anxiety, a daily dose of 2,000 mg of calcium and 1,000 mg of magnesium is probably optimum.

Potassium is necessary for a healthy nervous system. It calms the heart and relieves muscle pain. It also is essential for proper functioning of your adrenal glands, which get a good workout during anxiety and panic attacks. Signs of potassium deficiency include nervousness, fatigue, fluctuations in heartbeat, glucose intolerance, insomnia, respiratory distress, and nausea. The ability to transfer nutrients through cell membranes declines with age, which could explain why older people suffer circulatory damage, lethargy, and weakness from insufficient potassium. Taking extra potassium (99 mg a day) or eating potassium-rich foods (discussed below) could help.

It's important to maintain a proper balance of magnesium, calcium, and phosphorus. If one of these minerals is present in excessive or insufficient amounts, you can expect adverse effects in your body. Although deficiencies of *phosphorus* are rare, they can lead to anxiety, fatigue, irregular breathing, irritability, numbness, skin sensitivity, trembling, weakness, and weight changes.

Zinc exerts a calming effect on your central nervous system. Although getting your nutrients via food is best, if you need to take a supplement, 50–80 mg daily is a safe amount. Do not exceed 100 mg daily from all supplements.

The best way to obtain nutrients is by eating foods rich in the substance. The best foods to eat to increase your *calcium* intake are salmon with bones, sardines, almonds, asparagus, blackstrap molasses, brewer's yeast (unless you are prone to yeast infections), broccoli, cabbage, carob, collards, dandelion greens, figs, filberts, kale, kelp, mustard greens, oats, prunes, sesame seeds, turnip greens, and watercress.

The best foods to eat to increase your *magnesium* intake are fish, including salmon, apples, green leafy vegetables, apricots, avocados, bananas, blackstrap molasses, brewer's yeast (unless you are prone to yeast infections), brown rice, cantaloupe, dulse (a type of seaweed available in health food stores), figs, garlic, grapefruit, lima beans, millet (found in health food stores), nuts, peaches, black-eyed peas, sesame seeds, soybeans (and soy products such as soy nuts, tempeh, soy "cheese," and soy "meats"), watercress, and whole-grain breads and cereals.

The best foods to eat to increase your *phosphorus* intake are asparagus, brewer's yeast (unless you are prone to yeast infections), eggs, fish, including salmon, garlic, legumes (peanuts, dried beans, and dried peas), nuts, seeds (sesame, sunflower, and pumpkin), and whole-grain breads and cereals.

The best foods to eat to increase your *potassium* intake are fish, fruit, legumes, vegetables, and whole-grain breads and cereals.

Good food sources of *zinc* are brewer's yeast (unless you're prone to yeast infections), dulse, egg yolks, fish, including sardines, kelp, legumes, lima beans, mushrooms, pecans, pumpkin seeds, seafood, soy lecithin, soybeans, sunflower seeds, and whole grain breads and cereals.

Vitamins

The B complex vitamins are known as the antistress vitamins because they help maintain normal nervous system function, help reduce anxiety, and have a calming effect on the nerves. Good food sources of B vitamins include asparagus, avocados, blackstrap molasses, broccoli, brown rice, brussels sprouts, cabbage, carrots, currants, dandelion greens, dates, dulse, eggs, seafood, kelp, kombu and nori (health food store items), legumes, lentils, mushrooms, molasses, nuts, peanuts, peas, potatoes, soybeans and soybean products, raisins, raw spinach, split peas, sunflower seeds, tomatoes, walnuts, watercress, wheat germ and whole-grain breads and cereals.

Vitamin C is necessary for the proper functioning of your stress-control adrenal glands and brain chemistry. This vitamin can decrease anxiety and is vital for dealing with stress. Good food sources of this vitamin are asparagus, avocados, beet greens, black currants, broccoli, brussels sprouts, cantaloupe, collards, dandelion greens, dulse, kale, mangoes, mustard greens, onions, papaya, green peas, sweet peppers, persimmons, pineapple, radishes, spinach (raw), strawberries, Swiss chard, tomatoes, turnip greens, and watercress.

Iron

Iron deficiency can increase the risk of panic attacks. One of the best ways to make sure you get enough iron is to cook with iron pots and pans. Good food sources of iron include eggs, fish, green leafy vegetables, whole-grain breads and cereals, almonds, avocados, beets, blackstrap molasses, brewer's yeast (unless you're prone to yeast infections), dates, dulse, kelp, kidney and lima beans, lentils, millet, peaches, pears, pumpkin, raisins, sesame seeds, soybeans and soybean products, and watercress.

Many individuals do not absorb the iron in iron supplements, but there is a product called Floradix Iron + Herbs (from Salus Haus) that allows you to assimilate the iron you need. You can find it (or order it) in health food stores.

▊ Foods Associated with Less Stress

A study of stress and dietary practices revealed that greater stress was associated with more fatty food intake, less fruit and vegetable intake, more snacking, and reduced likelihood of daily breakfast consumption. These findings suggest that to reduce your anxiety, eat more fruits and vegetables and don't skip breakfast.

Another study found that omega-3 fatty acids reduced stress and anxiety. Omega-3 fatty acids are found in fatty fish such as salmon (arctic, free-range) and tuna (chunk light), fish oil capsules, flaxseed, canola oil, and walnuts. Two servings of fish a week will not only reduce anxiety but is recommended by the American Heart Association to reduce the risk of coronary heart disease. In an interesting study, populations from seven different world regions were studied for twenty-five years. Research teams found that eating fish, vegetables, legumes, olive oil, and a moderate intake of wine (all part of the Mediterranean diet) were associated with low rates of heart and blood vessel diseases. The same effects were found among those eating a diet rich in soy, cereals, and fish (the Asian diet).

Findings from another study suggest that selenium may affect your mood as well as your health. Individuals with low dietary intakes of selenium report feeling more anxious, depressed, and tired. Be sure to eat plenty of fish, shellfish, whole-grain breads and cereals, mushrooms, and Brazil nuts. You can also take an additional 150 to 200 micrograms (mcg) daily of selenium in the form of selenomethionine or selenium yeast.

Green tea has the ability to stimulate your brain in the same way deep meditation does. Besides calming you, it can also help you focus. This substance stimulates production of alpha waves in your brain, similar to what happens during deep meditation. It has the unique ability to make you feel calm but focused, so that your learning ability is enhanced. An amino acid (precursor to protein) found in the leaves of green tea and certain mushrooms called L-theanine compares favorably to Ativan, a synthetic tranquilizer that interferes with your ability to drive, is addictive, and can end up worsening anxiety as well as causing abnormal liver function. L-theanine is taken in 100 to 200 mg capsules two to three times day, but should be avoided by pregnant and nursing mothers, as it has not been studied on these women. If you want to drink green tea instead, the equivalent is 2–8 cups. Start with 2 cups and evaluate the effect before increasing your intake.

Moving toward a vegetarian dietary regime can also lower your anxiety, according to the results of a study that investigated the different kinds of diet and the levels of anxiety and depression participants aged twenty-five to seventy years reported. More anxiety and depression were reported in the nonvegetarian groups than in the vegetarian groups. Diet analysis also found more stress-reducing antioxidants in the vegetarian group than in the nonvegetarian group. These findings suggest that a diet focused primarily on vegetables, fruits, and grains is associated with less anxiety than a diet focused on meat or other animal products.

How can a vegetarian diet reduce anxiety? Meat, poultry, dairy foods, sugar, and refined-flour products are all acid-forming foods that leave an acid residue in the body after being metabolized. So do many medications. When your body is more acid, transit time of food is speeded up which results in underabsorption of vitamins, especially the stress vitamins (B and C) and minerals that reduce stress and make you feel more sluggish and fatigued. Unfortunately, merely taking additional vitamins and minerals usually will not correct this condition unless you also change your eating and medicating patterns so you can better absorb nutrients.

To attain a proper acid-alkaline balance in your body, eat more vegetables and fruits (except plums and prunes), whole grains (especially brown rice, millet, and buckwheat), and bean sprouts. Aim to get 70 percent of your calories from these foods, except in winter, when you may wish to eat a slightly higher percentage of animal protein.

Also make soy and soy products the main source of your protein. Research has shown that soy protects your nervous system. Using soy from organically produced (not genetically altered) foods has the potential for protecting and balancing your emotions and will not tip your body into acid imbalance.

Increasing your intake of certain amino acids may enhance your mood and behavior. Amino acids are the building blocks of protein. You can purchase amino acids individually in a health food store (as supplements), but this isn't recommended since they are meant to complement each other and you can't be sure how much to take to balance an imbalance. It's better to eat foods high in glutamine to treat fatigue and enhance mental functioning (eat more raw spinach and raw parsley), histidine to increase pleasure (eat more rice, wheat, and rye), methionine to enhance muscle strength (eat more beans, eggs, fish, garlic, lentils, onions, soybeans, seeds, and yogurt), taurine to reduce heart palpitations (eat more eggs, fish, meat), tryptophan to combat depression and insomnia and stabilize mood (eat more cheese, turkey, brown rice, cottage cheese, and soy protein.)

To obtain a balanced amount of all amino acids, you can use Bragg Liquid Aminos (a health food store item). It's made from soy and looks and tastes like soy sauce. You can use it in soups, stews, salad dressing, on vegetables, and in dips.

Supplements to Reduce Anxiety

Vitamin C (ascorbic acid) may help reduce anxiety. It decreases stress reactivity and can help you stay calm. A vitamin and mineral supplement may also be helpful. One study examined the relative effectiveness of a vitamin and mineral supplement and a placebo (sugar pill). The researchers found that as compared to placebo, the supplement was associated with significant reductions in anxiety and perceived stress. Lysine is another supplement that has been shown to reduce chronic anxiety and lessen stress. Many people find some relief at 500 mg a day.

If you're anxious, it could be because you have a B-vitamin and magnesium deficiency. B vitamins (as well as vitamin C) are rapidly depleted during stressful and anxiety-ridden situations. All these supplements are relatively safe, have few side effects, and are low in cost.

Gamma-aminobutyric acid (GABA) is an amino acid (protein precursor) that acts as a neurotransmitter in your central nervous system and is formed in the body from another amino acid, glutamic acid. GABA inhibits nerve cells from overfiring. Together with niacinamide and inositol (two B vitamins) they prevent anxiety- and stress-related messages from reaching your brain.

GABA can be taken to calm you in much the same way as a tranquilizer, but without fear of addiction. Note that if you take too much it can increase anxiety and make you short of breath, numb around the mouth, and tingly in the extremities. A helpful level is 750 mg twice a day.

Chromium deficiency can produce anxiety symptoms. Daily take 200 mcg.

The amino acid L-glutamine has a mild tranquilizing effect. Take it on an empty stomach at a dose of 500 mg three times a day. Never take it with milk. Use water or juice, and for better absorption add 50 mg vitamin B_6 and 100 mg of vitamin C.

Another amino acid, L-tyrosine, may also relieve anxiety and depression, but avoid this supplement if you are taking an MAO-inhibitor drug. The usual dose is 500 mg three times a day on an empty stomach. Consider taking it in concert with L-glycine (500 mg three times daily) on an empty stomach.

Stressless Eating

The way you eat can also increase your anxiety. It doesn't matter what you eat if you don't eat in a calm manner that aids digestion. To reduce your anxiety, slow down your eating process. Use the following guidelines:

- Avoid doing anything else while eating.
- Always sit down when eating; never eat "on the run."
- Chew everything well before swallowing. Focus on the smell, taste, look, and sensation of each food.
- Avoid overeating. This can stress your body, make for foggy thinking, and lead to obesity, which can also increase anxiety.
- Avoid drinking cold or iced fluids while eating; they stress your digestive track and dilute digestive enzymes.

▊ Summary of Self-Care Actions

Take these steps to reduce your level of anxiety:

Avoid:
1. caffeine (including medications that contain caffeine)
2. salt
3. nicotine
4. sugar
5. alcohol (see chapter 7)
6. meat, dairy products, and any animal products
7. stressful eating (eating on the run, skipping meals, overeating, insufficient chewing, multitasking while eating, cold or iced drinks)

Focus On:

1. whole fruits and vegetables, preferably organic (no pesticides or steroids)
2. whole-grain cereals, breads, and pastas
3. soy products (soy cheese, soy meats, soy nuts, tempeh; but avoid tofu that has been produced in aluminum pans)
4. fish (especially fatty varieties, such as chunk light tuna, and arctic salmon) and flaxseeds (find in the health food store; make into a powder in blender and add to soups, salads, juices, water, and cereals)
5. walnuts
6. olive and canola oils
7. stress tabs (C and B-complex vitamins)
8. lysine (find in a health food store and follow directions on the bottle; better yet, eat lysine-rich foods, such as eggs, fish, lima beans, potatoes, and soy products)
9. chromium: take as chromium picolinate, 200 mcg/day; better yet, eat brewer's yeast (unless you are susceptible to yeast infections), brown rice, whole grains (breads, cereals, pastas), dried beans, blackstrap molasses, corn, eggs, mushrooms, and potatoes
10. a daily vitamin and mineral supplement
11. stressless eating

6

Herbs

Many herbs contain minerals and vitamins and are one way to ingest these needed nutrients.

Bob, a fifty-two-year-old executive, had struggled with anxiety for years. He tried to change his eating plan but failed. He started taking calcium, magnesium, and potassium supplements, but they didn't agree with him. When he started drinking herbal teas that contained minerals, he finally found a method that worked for him.

The vitamin-mineral table below shows which herbs supply which nutrients.

Vitamin-Mineral Table		
Herbs	**Vitamins**	**Minerals**
alfalfa, bladderwrack, burdock catnip, cayenne, chamomile, chickweed, eyebright, fennel, fenugreek, hops, nettle, oat straw,		

Herbs	Vitamins	Minerals
parsley, peppermint, raspberry leaf, red clover, rose hips, sage, yarrow, and yellow dock	B_1 (thiamine)	
alfalfa, bladderwrack, burdock, catnip, cayenne, chamomile, chickweed, eyebright, fennel seed, fenugreek, ginseng, hops, horsetail, mullein, nettle, oat straw, parsley, peppermint, raspberry leaf, red clover, rose hips, sage, and yellow dock	B_2 (riboflavin)	
alfalfa, burdock, catnip, cayenne, chamomile, chickweed, eyebright, fennel, hops, licorice, mullein, nettle, oat straw, parsley, peppermint, raspberry leaf, red clover, rose hips, slippery elm, and yellow dock	B_3 (Niacin)	
alfalfa, catnip, and oat straw	B_6 (Pyridoxine)	
alfalfa, bladderwrack, and hops	B_{12} (cyanocobalamin)	
alfalfa, burdock, cayenne, chickweed, eyebright, fennel seed, fenugreek, hops, horsetail, peppermint, mullein, nettle, oat straw, paprika, parsley, plantain, raspberry leaf, red clover, rose hips, skullcap, violet leaves, yarrow, and yellow dock	vitamin C	
alfalfa, horsetail, nettle, and parsley	vitamin D	
alfalfa, bladderwrack, dandelion, dong quai, flaxseed, nettle, oat straw, raspberry leaf, and rose hips	vitamin E	
alfalfa, green tea, kelp, nettle, oat straw, and shepherd's purse	vitamin K	

Herbs	Vitamins	Minerals
chervil, elderberries, hawthorn berry, horsetail, rose hips, and shepherd's purse	bioflavonoids	
alfalfa, burdock, cayenne, chamomile, chickweed, chickory, dandelion, eyebright, fennel seed, fenugreek, flaxseed, hops, horsetail, kelp, lemongrass, plantain, raspberry leaf, red clover, rose hips, shepherd's purse, violet leaves, yarrow, and yellow dock		calcium
catnip, horsetail, licorice, nettle, oat straw, red clover, sarsaparilla, wild yam, and yarrow		chromium
alfalfa, burdock, catnip, cayenne, chamomile, chickweed, chicory, dandelion, dong quai, eyebright, fennel seed, fenugreek, horsetail, kelp, lemongrass, licorice, milk thistle seed, mullein, nettle, oat straw, paprika, parsley, peppermint, plantain, raspberry leaf, rose hips, sarsaparilla, shepherd's purse, uva ursi, and yellow dock		iron
alfalfa, bladderwrack, catnip, cayenne, chamomile, chickweed, dandelion, eyebright, fennel seed, fenugreek, hops, horsetail, lemongrass, licorice, mullein, nettle, oat straw, paprika, parsley, peppermint, raspberry leaf, red clover, sage, shepherd's purse, yarrow, and yellow dock		magnesium
alfalfa, burdock, catnip, chamomile, chickweed, dandelion, eyebright, fennel seed, fenugreek, ginseng,		

Herbs	Vitamins	Minerals
hops, horsetail, lemongrass, mullein, parsley, peppermint, raspberry leaf, red clover, rose hips, wild yam, yarrow, and yellow dock		manganese
catnip, hops, horsetail, nettle, plantain, red clover, sage, and skullcap		potassium
alfalfa, burdock, catnip, cayenne, chamomile, chickweed, fennel seed, fenugreek, garlic, ginseng, hawthorn berry, hops, horsetail, lemongrass, milk thistle, nettle, oat straw, parsley, peppermint, raspberry leaf, rose hips, sarsaparilla, uva ursi, yarrow, and yellow dock		selenium
horsetail		sulfur
alfalfa, burdock, cayenne, chamomile, chickweed, dandelion, eyebright, fennel seed, hops, milk thistle, mullein, nettle, parsley, rose hips, sage, sarsaparilla, skullcap, and wild yam		zinc

∎ The Benefits of Herbs

Herbs offer an effective but gentle approach to the physiological and chemical issues involved in anxiety reduction. They support the adrenal glands and ease the many symptoms associated with anxiety. In most cases they work more quickly than tranquilizers.

Herbs are used for a wide range of anxious symptoms, including worry, apprehension, anticipation of the worst, and irritability. Relaxant herbs treat symptoms, and should never be used to mask a systemic problem. If stress is a way of life for you, relaxant herbs are only part of the answer.

If you decide to try one of these herbs, many can be purchased as teas or in bulk. Start with 1 teaspoon of herb per cup of boiling water and steep for 5–15 minutes. Drink ½ cup three times a day. If necessary, work up to 1 cup three times a day. If you prefer to take capsules, search out a standardized form and follow the directions on the label.

Always tell your health-care practitioner what herbs you are considering or are already taking. If you experience any symptoms, always stop taking the herb and report your reaction to your health-care practitioner. Never stop taking a prescribed drug without discussing it with your health-care practitioner. Purchase a herb book and/or work with a herbalist if you plan to use herbs. Though more gentle than many drugs they are still powerful substances.

Sarah, a thirty-two-year-old yoga instructor, had tried several herbs for her anxiety, including chamomile, motherwort, and valerian, but had not achieved total calmness. When she found a Chinese formula bupleurum and started taking it regularly, her anxiety decreased and her feelings of well-being increased.

This client exemplifies why no specific herbs are recommended in this chapter. Different herbs work well for some individuals and not for others. You may have to experiment and try an herb for a week or two to see which one works for you. Some herbs are easily found. For example, Celestial Seasonings chamomile is available in supermarkets. Other herbs, such as many of the Chinese herbs, are only available in Chinese markets or from Chinese medicine herbalists. In some cases, you may need to inquire at a health food or herbal store to find specific herbs. Always start with a small amount, observe for any changes, and only gradually increase the amount over days, and only if needed.

Albizzia Bark

Albizzia is a Chinese herb that is prescribed for emotional problems. It has a neutral energy and is sweet tasting. The bark is calming and improves mood. It helps with anxiety, insomnia, irritability, anger, and excessive worry.

Ashwaganda

Ashwaganda is an ayurvedic herb. In one study, individuals who had been diagnosed with anxiety disorders were given ashwaganda. In most cases, participants' mental condition improved in three months.

Blue Vervain

This flower is a herb known as a nervine or nerve tonic; it is sedative and antispasmodic (stops muscle spasms). These attributes make it useful for reducing anxiety and nervousness. It soothes and relaxes the nervous system, helps with insomnia and nervous stomach. To drink as a tea, put ½ teaspoon of the herb in a cup of water and take ½ cup of tea three times daily. If taking the tincture, use 30 drops or ¼ teaspoon three times a day (for children, halve this amount and sweeten with honey).

Biota Seed

Biota is another Chinese herb. It is most commonly used in Chinese tonics. It has a neutral energy and a sweet taste. It is calming and sedative and can be used to reduce fear, anxiety, and insomnia.

Bupleurum Formula

This Chinese tonic is used to inhibit excitability due to an over-abundance of liver energy (*qi*). The liver, believed to be the seat of nerves in the Chinese system of healing, is sedated, resulting in calmness. This formula is commonly used to treat irritability, chronic anger, nervousness, hysteria, tension, spasms, tremors, insomnia due to excitability, grinding of the teeth during sleep, severe neck tension, and spasms due to nervous tension.

Catnip

Studies show catnip is good not only for cats. German researchers report that the chemicals responsible for cats' intoxication (nepetalactone isomers) are similar to the natural sedatives in valerian (valepotriates). This finding supports catnip's traditional use as a mild tranquilizer and sedative. Try a cup of tea when you feel tense or before bed to see if this herb works for you.

Chamomile

Chamomile is used to soothe and relax during the daytime. Because it's a mild relaxant, it's not usually used as a sleep aid. Chamomile is superior to many tranquilizers because it does not disrupt normal performance or function but reduces anxiety.

Take chamomile as a tea. It is a refreshing, sweet beverage. Do not take if you're allergic to flowers.

Dragon Bone

This sweet and astringent Chinese herb has a strong calming effect, which is both sedating and relaxing. It is known for calming excitability and has been used to treat insomnia, restlessness, apprehension, palpitations, anxiety, irritability, anger, frustration, tension, and fear. It is extremely safe.

Gotu Kola

Although gota kola has many uses, including healing wounds and improving circulation to the legs, it also relieves anxiety and promotes sleep. Because this herb can result in a skin rash, it's important to talk with a health-care practitioner familiar with this herb and its uses. The dosage is two to four 400 mg capsules a day of *H. asiatica*, the least expensive form of gotu kola.

Kava-Kava Root

The dried roots of kava-kava are used in Polynesia to calm (in small doses) or induce sleep. A dose of 1 ounce of the herb in tea or capsules (up to 280 mg a day) is safe. Kava-kava costs about one-tenth the price of Xanax, doesn't impair reaction time or concentration as do antianxiety drugs like Xanax and actually improves mental function; it does not promote sedation, does not lose effectiveness over time as drugs do, and has no side effects when taken at recommended doses (47 to 70 mg of kavalactones three times daily). The German Commission E (the government health agency that publishes monographs on herbs) states that kava-kava should not be used during pregnancy, while breast-feeding, or if you are depressed or have liver damage.

Although there was an uproar about the dangers of this herb several years ago, the research findings continue to show it is safe unless you have the above-listed conditions.

Linden Flowers

The tea made from linden flowers has been used since the Middle Ages to reduce anxiety, invigorate the mind, and soothe the body. Some research has shown that continued frequent use of linden flower tea can damage the heart. In therapeutic doses, especially in capsules (follow the label), linden is nontoxic.

Motherwort

The ancient Greeks and Romans used motherwort for both physical and emotional problems of the heart—palpitations and depression. European colonists introduced motherwort into North America and prescribed it as a tranquilizer for nervous excitement, restlessness, and disturbed sleep. German studies show motherwort has a mild sedative effect, comparable to valerian, making it useful for anxiety and insomnia. Try two cups of tea a day with honey (it is bitter) or ½ to 1 teaspoon as a tincture twice a day. Should not be given to children below the age of two.

Nutmeg

Nutmeg can also be used to bring on sleep and may even be more powerful than valerian. The herb must be taken four to five hours prior to sleep, but once it takes hold, sleep lasts for eight hours, so it is more effective to keep you sleeping than valerian. For best results, whole nutmeg should be freshly ground in a coffee grinder or blender and then placed in capsules.

Because of its power, start with 1 capsule four to five hours before bedtime and take another if you don't get the effect you want. To stay relaxed throughout the day, you can take another one in the morning.

Passion Flower

Like valerian, passion flower has a long history of being used as a sedative, or nervine, to combat anxiety and nervousness, to end muscle cramps, to tranquilize, and to induce sleep. Passion flower was discovered in Peru by the Spanish doctor Monardes in 1569 and is now used worldwide. Research has shown that passion flower preparations overcome nervous symptoms and cramps that inhibit sleep and produce a restful and deep sleep free from frequent awakenings. It sedates the central nervous system, helping overcome anxiety and nervousness.

Passion flower is not toxic and has no side effects. The herb has been approved by the Food and Drug Administration for food use. There are no known contraindications for passion flower, but use whole-plant preparations, not isolated alkaloids, which can be hallucinogenic.

Pearl

Pearl is a tonic herb that is used in the Orient as an antistress supplement. It can relieve uneasiness, nervousness, anxiety, and tension. It also promotes sound sleep, prevents nervous disorders and nerve weakness, and overcomes fatigue. Consistent use can help maintain energy and vitality. Safety studies have shown pearl to be absolutely harmless, and it can be taken indefinitely by anybody without side effects.

Peppermint Leaf

This herb contains several essential oils that prevent congestion of the blood supply to the brain, stimulate and clear circulation, and strengthen and calm nerves, creating a calming effect. Take as a tea after meals to aid in digestion and relax the mind and body.

Rosemary Leaf

Rosemary—yes, the same rosemary you probably use to spice up your lamb dish—contains valuable essential oils that calm and soothe irritated nerves and upset stomachs, and extinguish anxiety. Rosemary is also very high in calcium, magnesium, phosphorus, sodium, and potassium, which are required by nerves and heart muscle for proper functioning.

Suanzaorentang

This Chinese formulation of zizyphi seed, ligustrum, licorice, poria, and bunge root known as suanzaorentang has proven almost as effective as the anti-anxiety drug Valium (diazepam) in dealing with anxiety, weakness, irritability, and insomnia. When taken three times a day, this herbal combination improves motor skills and produces none of the side effects of Valium. In a European study this Chinese formulation helped individuals with severe anxiety attacks, including chest pain, shortness of breath, and heart palpitations.

Valerian Root

Valerian is a short-term sedative that works in two weeks, whereas drugs can take six weeks to take effect. In one study, individuals with anxiety and depression took hops and valerian, which took effect in two weeks and caused far fewer side effects than prescription drugs.

Valerian is at least as effective as Valium and Xanax, but is not habit forming and does not interact with other drugs or alcohol the way prescription tranquilizers do. An overdose of Valerian results only in headache and mild tremors that resolve in twenty-four hours, while taking Valium with alcohol can cause death.

In Europe, Valerian is widely used instead of Valium or Xanax for anxiety. More than 200 studies showing the herb's effectiveness have been conducted there, and the herb is likely to be recommended by physicians instead of pharmaceuticals. Prior to the 1940s and the rise of the pharmaceutical industry, valerian was used to relax muscles. Research has also shown it to be effective with hyperactive children, but don't use the herb with children (or pregnant or nursing women) except on the advice of a knowledgeable health practitioner.

If insomnia is a problem for you, consider taking valerian root. It offers a healthy, nontoxic alternative to prescription drugs; it works best if you have trouble falling asleep, but it does not increase the quality of sleep. Valerian can also be used to withdraw from an addiction to sleeping pills.

Because of the acrid smell of brewed valerian root tea, the best way to take valerian is either as a capsule, tablet, or tincture. It may take five to ten capsules or tablets to get the desired effect. Two tablets or capsules may calm your nerves, but more may be needed for sleep. Start with two and work up until you obtain the desired result.

■ Summary

1. Discuss your plans to use herbs with your health-care practitioner.
2. Never just discontinue taking a prescribed drug and switch to herbs; work out a schedule with your health-care practitioner.
3. Never take more of a herb than is recommended.
4. Don't use herbs with children, or pregnant or nursing women, except on the advice of a knowledgeable health-care practitioner.
5. If you plan to use herbs, purchase a herb book or work with a herbalist. Herbs are potent substances and should only be used by a well-informed person.

7

Environmental Changes

You may not even think about your environment as a source of anxiety, but it can be.

Sally, a part-time data processor and single mother of twins, smoked two packs a day and drank a bottle of wine after her four-year-olds went to bed. She had started drinking just a glass or two of wine, but as time rolled on, she found she had to keep upping the amount to get the same results she used to get on a smaller amount of alcohol. Without her wine, Sally had a hard time getting to sleep. During the day, her hands shook and she felt anxious. She spent little time outside in the fresh air. Her office had poor ventilation and too much humidity, and so did her house. When she started to refinish furniture at home, her anxiety level doubled.

■ Unnatural Environments and Anxiety

Polluted and other unnatural environments can lead to anxiety. The following are some of the major environmental conditions that you can control.

Nicotine

A recent study tied heavy smoking to agoraphobia, generalized anxiety disorder, and panic disorder. Of adolescents who smoked heavily, 31 percent developed anxiety disorders in adulthood. Another study found that smoking increased the risk of panic. Being around smokers and smoky conditions can also affect you.

Nicotine is a strong stimulant that constricts blood vessels and makes your heart work harder. Although smokers believe that having a cigarette "calms their nerves," research has shown that smokers are more anxious and sleep less well than nonsmokers. Quitting smoking not only leads to fewer panic attacks and lower levels of anxiety but to better health and vitality.

Here are some tips for quitting smoking that you (or your family members) can use:

1. Ask yourself, *"What is this habit doing for me?"* (It's doing something or you wouldn't keep it!)
2. Ask yourself, *"What is this habit costing me?"*
3. *Decide* how you could get these things without using so much negative energy.
4. *Write your plan for* what you will do today to stop smoking. *(Join a group or find a supportive buddy to work along with you.)*
5. *Eat more* fruits, vegetables, and grains. Eat half a grapefruit after a meal to reduce the urge to smoke and then brush your teeth.

6. *Avoid* caffeinated drinks that increase craving for cigarettes, and alcohol, which decreases your willpower.

7. *Drink* eight glasses of water a day and avoid beverages with a lot of calories—sodas, juices, and milk—that can add weight.

8. *Get rid of* all cigarettes and ashtrays in your home, car, and workplace.

9. *Ask* your family, friends, and coworkers for support.

10. *Stay in nonsmoking areas.*

11. *Breathe in deeply and wait five minutes* (by the clock) whenever you feel the urge to smoke. (Second month, increase the wait to ten minutes; third month increase to fifteen minutes.)

12. *Keep yourself busy.* Hold something in your hand other than a cigarette—e.g., cinnamon stick, toothpick, pen or pencil, straw. Take up a hobby that occupies your hands—e.g., knitting, crocheting, painting, playing an instrument, writing. Cut up raw vegetables and have one, or chew a piece of gum, when you have an urge to smoke.

13. *Reward yourself often*, especially by planning a present for yourself with the money you save from not smoking.

14. *Set a quit date (in writing) and stick to it.* Quitting cold turkey is best and is associated with the fewest withdrawal symptoms. (Physical addiction to nicotine lasts only forty-eight hours—you can do it!)

15. *Learn relaxation skills* (see chapter 9).

16. *Do at least one enjoyable activity every day.*

17. *Remind yourself of the rewards of quitting*: your health will improve; food will taste better, and your sense of smell will improve; you'll save money and feel better about yourself; home/car/breath will smell better; you can stop worrying about quitting; you'll be setting a good example for others, and you'll have no more worries about

exposing others to smoke; free from addiction, you'll feel better physically, and perform better at sports.

18. *Start an exercise program and follow it.*
19. *Reduce your exposure to smoke.* If anyone in your household smokes, that puts you at risk for osteoporosis. Try to convince that person to quit. If you can't, insist that they smoke outside the house only.

Alcohol

Alcohol can increase anxiety and even precipitate panic attacks. People with anxiety may drink to reduce anxiety, but down the road alcohol takes over and creates even more anxiety. Even moderate drinking can complicate or compromise anxiety treatment. Sometimes just avoiding alcohol can reduce anxiety.

Denial is a major problem for people who abuse alcohol or are dependent on it. Besides claiming drinking isn't a problem for you, you may employ minimizing ("I drink, but it's not a problem"; "It's no big deal"; "I made it home in one piece, so it can't be that bad"), blaming ("I need to drink because of how bad my life is"; "I need to drink to put up with other people"; "My family drives me to drink"; "It wasn't my fault for getting drunk"), stonewalling ("I can quit any time I want"; "It's my business how much I drink"; "I'm not hurting anyone but myself"; "I can handle my liquor"), excusing ("Alcohol helps me relax"; "I only need a drink to steady my nerves"; "I'm okay because I can still do what I have to do"; "This isn't a hangover, I have the flu"; "Everyone in my family drank"; "I'm under a lot of stress"), attacking ("Get off my back"; "Stop nagging"; "I'll stop drinking when you stop smoking"; "You've got some nerve telling me what to do"), rationalizing ("I'm already loaded, so one more won't make any difference"; "I need a lift when I'm down"; "I like living on the edge"; "I'll quit tomorrow"; "I deserve a reward"; "A nightcap will help me get a good night's sleep"), or distracting ("You'd drink too if you had to put up with what I have to"; "Alcohol is only a symptom of my screwed-up life").

If you answer "yes" to any of the next three questions, you probably have a drinking problem even though you may not think so.

1. Has anybody ever told you that you drink too much?
2. Do other people have a different opinion of your drinking than you do?
3. Do you sometimes think that alcohol is causing a problem in your life?

If you have most of the following danger signs, your drinking is serious and you need to quit:

1. You drink too much or too often.
2. Alcohol has endangered your life, relationships, job, schoolwork, or freedom.
3. You can't keep promises to yourself about your use of alcohol.
4. During the past twelve months you've been arrested for driving while intoxicated.
5. You suffer withdrawal symptoms when you try to stop drinking.
6. Your tolerance level has increased, so it takes more alcohol to get you high or achieve the desired effect.

When Sally looked at the various forms of denial, she had to admit she used distracting, rationalizing, and attacking. She decided she wanted to take action to reduce her drinking because it was making her more and more anxious and becoming more and more of a problem. We discussed joining a twelve-step program, where she could get help in avoiding high-risk situations, expressing her feelings, improving communication skills, and making amends.

Chemical Contaminants

When the air you breathe is full of contaminants, it can decrease your well-being and lead to discomfort and anxiety. This mix of pollutants can be transformed as a consequence of chemical reactions that can affect comfort and health.

Some of the contaminants you might be exposed to include:

1. formaldehyde (released from formaldehyde-based insulation foams and resin glues used in wood composition boards)
2. volatile organic compounds (benzene, naphtha, toluene, and many others released from solvents, paints, waxes, cleaners, upholstery, and plastics)
3. plasticizers (phthalates added to plastics to keep them soft and which have the "new" smell of a new auto interior, shower curtain, or plastic upholstery)
4. electromagnetic fields (from radio, TV, and microwave transmitters and high-voltage electrical lines; computers, televisions, and microwave ovens emit small amounts and should not be used close to the body)
5. bacteria and fungi (survive and reproduce at our body temperature; at humidities below 30 percent they will dry the protective mucous membranes of the throat and sinuses; at humidities above 60 percent they will grow on any organic material (including soil, food, wood, dust, resins, fibers, and urea formaldehyde foam)

Lack of Time-Management Skills

Signs of inappropriate time management include rushing, fatigue, chronic vacillation between unpleasant alternatives, chronic missing of deadlines, insufficient time allowed for rest or personal relationships, and the sense of being overwhelmed by demands and details.

Eloise exemplified most of these signs. She told me she never had enough time to achieve her goals and always rushed from one poor choice to another, always with a sense of feeling overwhelmed. At work she never met deadlines and was always asking for extensions. She complained of always feeling tired and never found enough time to rest and revive.

▮ Anti-Anxiety Actions

You can change your environment to make it less anxiety-provoking. Here are some suggestions.

Aromatherapy

Aromatherapy is the use of essential oils—fragrant, concentrated extracts of plants—to reduce symptoms and promote relaxation. Essential oils can be applied on your body, incorporated into ointments and compresses, inhaled, or taken internally to reduce anxiety. When compared to humidified air alone, heliotropin (a vanilla-like scent) was associated with 63 percent less anxiety in one study.

Almost all essential oils should be diluted in a vegetable carrier oil such as sweet almond, jojoba, or safflower oil before using to calm frazzled nerves and reduce anxiety. Mix together equal parts of lavender, geranium, ylang-ylang, and bergamot in a five-milliliter bottle. When you feel anxious, use 50 drops of this blend in a diffuser (which reduces essential oils to a fine spray and disperses the scent throughout the room), a scent ring (which sits on a warm light bulb), or an aroma lamp (a porcelain or clay pot in which essential oils are mixed with water and heated over a candle). You can also add 6 drops to a hot bath, stirring to disperse, then relax in the water. Find essential oils and aromatherapy tools at your local health food store.

Biofeedback

Biofeedback is a process for getting feedback from your body about internal processes. Breathing with awareness, using imagery, and employing any intervention that gives you feedback about your body are included in biofeedback.

More specifically, the word *biofeedback* is used to refer to the use of instrumentation to develop the ability to read tension in various body systems. Instruments are especially useful when you can't identify signs of anxiety, such as decreased hand temperature, increased muscle tension, or increased blood pressure.

Biofeedback instruments monitor your body via electrodes that detect internal changes and transform them into a visual or auditory signal, such as a sound, a flickering light, or readings on a meter. Anxiety, insomnia, muscle spasm or pain, teeth grinding, and other symptoms have been treated by biofeedback. You can go to a biofeedback practitioner or purchase your own inexpensive monitoring equipment for home use. Results may be better if you work with a highly trained and certified practitioner who can help you to overcome any roadblocks that might interrupt your progress.

Music

Recorded music has been studied and found effective in reducing anxiety. Music can affect your mood. It can make you feel relaxed, excited, comforted, and more. But music has even more extraordinary power. It can heal you. Particular sounds, rhythms, and tones, and especially the music of Mozart, Gregorian chant, some jazz, and New Age music, can reduce anxiety.

At the University of Massachusetts Medical Center, patients are encouraged to listen to soothing music and to perform relaxation exercises and meditation. This innovative program was developed by Jon Kabat-Zinn, director of the stress reduction and relaxation program, and harpist Georgia Kelly. It offers a safe, natural alternative to tranquilizers and other mood-altering drugs.

Jeanne Acterberg, PhD, pioneer in transpersonal psychology, imagery, and shamanic healing, used music in her own healing process after surgery; she found particular value in Mozart's "Laudate Dominum," from the CD *Cosmic Classics*.

Try different types of music and see what is soothing for you. Start with Beethoven and Mozart and experiment.

Natural Household Products

Synthetic products can create and add to anxiety and increase palpitations. The table below suggests some healthy environmental materials and additional alternatives to use if you can't find the items in the Healthy Materials column.

Component	Healthy Materials	Alternatives
area rugs, hangings	light-colored untreated cotton	untreated wool, acetate, or linen
bedding	untreated cotton mattress, cover, blankets	untreated wool or acetate materials
clothes	cotton, silk, linen, or wool	
doors	hollow-core metal	hardwood
finishes	bare plaster, casein	nonpetroleum-based finishes
fixtures, trims	metals, solid hardwoods	
floors	ceramic tile set in cement mortar	hardwood strip or plank
furniture frames	metal or solid hardwoods	
house frame	lightweight steel	softwood lumber
insulation	untreated mineral wood or glass fiber sealed by tight air/vapor tape	

Component	Healthy Materials	Alternatives
lamps	glass and metal only, certified totally enclosed	ventilated, recessed ceiling conventional fixtures of metal or glass, compact fluorescents
paints and varnishes	milk-based paint	self-tested acceptable paint, sealers, and varnishes
walls	untreated plaster, expanded metal lath, brick or concrete	untreated plaster on gypsum lath, hardwoods
windows	bare metal sash with well-cured plain silicone glass settings	enameled metal, hardwood

Sunlight

Research has shown that sunlight can relieve anxiety and depression. Aim for fifteen minutes a day in the sunshine with your face and arms exposed. Sitting outside and eating lunch or a snack is one way to do this. So is taking a short walk during lunchtime.

Time-Management Skills

The first step to better time management is to *explore how time is currently being spent*. An easy way to do this is to divide the day into three segments: waking through lunch, end of lunch through dinner, and end of dinner until bedtime. Carry around a small notebook and jot down the number of minutes you spend for each activity undertaken. Keep an inventory for three days, then total the amount of time you spend in each segments.

Here's a sample of Eloise's inventory:

Activity	Time	Activity	Time
Waking Through Lunch		*After Lunch Through Dinner*	
lying in bed, thinking about getting up	20 minutes	attend nonmandatory lecture	60 minutes
		working with clients	90 minutes
showering	20 minutes	daydreaming while staring at paperwork	20 minutes
decide what to wear and get dressed	25 minutes	staff meeting	45 minutes
cook breakfast	15 minutes	socialize	30 minutes
read paper and eat	30 minutes	commute	30 minutes
phone friend	15 minutes	shop	45 minutes
commute to work	30 minutes	cook	90 minutes
routine paperwork	30 minutes	eat	30 minutes
nonmandatory meeting	60 minutes		
		After Dinner Until Retiring	
work with clients	120 minutes	phone calls	60 minutes
lunch	45 minutes	television	90 minutes
		Study	90 minutes
		prepare for bed/read	30 minutes

Your next step is to *make decisions about what can be cut out of your day.* Here are some of Eloise's choices.

- put out clothes for the next day prior to going to bed
- get up at the alarm and limit showering to 5 minutes
- make breakfasts that don't require cooking; cut dinner preparation to 30 minutes and enlist family to do food preparation and cleanup

- ask for a late lunch to take advantage of most productive work hours (11 A.M. to 2 P.M.)
- stop attending nonmandatory, nonproductive meetings
- use thought stopping (see chapter 9) to limit daydreaming and gossiping

Next, *set priorities*. Make a list of things you most want to accomplish in the near future and compare it to how you currently spend your time. Visualize yourself being told you only have six months left to live and plan how you'd spend your time.

Choose goals. Make a list of one-month, one-year, and lifetime goals. Make sure they're reasonable. Decide which goals are top-drawer (most essential or desired), middle-drawer (important, but can be put off for a while), and bottom-drawer (can be put off indefinitely with no harm done).

Here are the top-drawer goals Eloise chose for her one-month, one-year, and lifetime goals (two of each):

1. Buy a new car. (one-year goal)
2. Write an article for a journal. (lifetime goal)
3. Have dinner out with husband once a week. (one-month goal)
4. Investigate ways of becoming a consultant. (lifetime goal)
5. Take dance lessons with husband. (one-year goal)
6. Complete paperwork. (one-month goal)

Since Eloise was overwhelmed by the six goals, she decided to break each one into manageable steps. For example, she decided her goal of investigating ways of becoming a consultant into the following steps:

1. Borrow a friend's book on consulting and read a chapter a week.

2. Talk with other women I know who are consultants and ask one or more to be my mentor.
3. Make a list of my knowledge and skills that would make me salable as a consultant.
4. Purchase stationary, business cards, and brochures detailing my consulting skills.

Eloise still found it difficult to get started even after breaking down her priorities into manageable steps, so she developed a daily "to do" list that included everything she wanted to accomplish that day. She rated each item top-, middle-, or bottom-priority for the day. This approach helped, but Eloise still needed to discover the rules for making time, including:

1. Learn to say no to others. Remind yourself that this is your life and that your time is your own, to spend as best benefits you. Only when your boss asks should you spend time on bottom-priority items. Be prepared to say, "I don't have the time." If necessary, take an assertiveness-training course to help you learn to say no.
2. Build time into your schedule for unscheduled events, interruptions, and unforeseen circumstances. Remember that things always take longer than you think they will.
3. Set aside several time periods during the day for structured relaxation. Being relaxed will allow you to use the time you have more efficiently.
4. Keep a list of short 5-minute tasks that can be completed anytime you are waiting or are between other tasks.
5. Learn to do two things at once; for example, plan dinner while driving home, or organize an important letter or list while waiting in line at the bank.
6. Delegate bottom-drawer tasks to sons, daughters, secretaries, or in-laws.

7. Get up 15 to 20 minutes earlier each day.

8. Allow no more than 1 hour of television-watching for yourself daily. Use TV as a reward for working on your top-drawer items.

Part of time management is the ability to make decisions. Procrastination is a great time robber. Here are some ways to overcome this time robber:

1. Compare the unpleasantness of making some decisions to the unpleasantness of putting them off. Analyze the costs and risks of delay.

2. Examine the payoffs you receive for procrastinating, such as not having to face the possibility of failure, being taken care of by others, getting attention by being chronically unhappy.

3. Exaggerate and intensify whatever you are doing to put off the decision. Keep it up until you're bored and making the decision seems more attractive than whatever you are doing to procrastinate.

4. Take responsibility for your delaying tactics by writing down how long each delay took.

5. When having trouble choosing between alternatives that have the same number of positives as negatives, choose south or east over north or west, pick left over right, smooth over rough, the shortest, the closest, or the one that comes first in the alphabet.

6. Take small steps toward a decision to get yourself ready. For example, if you decide to sew on a button, take out the thread and materials and place them by you as a lead-in to the decision to begin.

7. Avoid beginning a new task until you have completed a predetermined segment of the current one.

▌ Summary

To reduce environmental sources of anxiety:

1. Stop smoking.
2. Stop drinking alcohol.
3. Avoid chemical contaminants.
4. Learn time-management skills.
5. Use aromatherapy.
6. Explore using biofeedback.
7. Use music.
8. Purchase natural household products.
9. Spend 15 minutes in the sun daily.

8

Exercise

Exercise can be a potent anti-anxiety measure because it can trig-ger release of "feel good" endorphins that help reduce anxiety and depression, and improve sleep and sexual activity. If you're not exercising and you suffer from anxiety, now is the time to consider starting a daily program.

Jackie, age twenty-eight, has been taking tranquilizers since ado-lescence. When she started line-dancing lessons because a man she was dating wanted her to go dancing with him, Jackie discov-ered a significant decrease in her anxiety after the first class. Be-cause every tranquilizer she tried resulted in uncomfortable side effects, Jackie focused on dancing and nutritional approaches to keep her anxiety in a reasonable comfort range.

■ How Exercise Affects Anxiety

Movement is one of the simplest and most effective ways to reduce anxiety and stress. It also moderates appetite, lowers cholesterol, reduces migraine, and slows aging. When done correctly, movement and exercise can enhance self-image and self-confidence, reduce muscle and joint stiffness, reduce depression, positively affect work performance, enhance ability to relate to others, enhance breathing ability, and improve the quality of sleep.

Exercise can be as potent as a tranquilizer in its effects, with none of the side effects, if you don't overdo it. In some cases, exercise may reduce your anxiety better than a counseling session.

Exercise is one of the most effective ways to reduce anxiety, and even panic attacks. Panic is simply the physical and emotional experience of an excessive surge of adrenaline. It is your body's "fight-or-flight" reaction gone wrong. Exercise provides a natural outlet for your body when you're exposed to too much adrenaline. Most of my clients who undertook a regular exercise program reported feeling less vulnerable to panic attacks and having less severe attacks when they did occur.

Exercising can take you out of the daily pressure of your life and help you focus on your body. This is important because much of anxiety occurs as a result of worry and repetitive negative thinking. When you are focusing on your body, you are not worrying or obsessing, which is why rest and meditation can also lead to relaxation. The difference between exercise and quiet rest or meditation is that after a fitness activity, the effect lasts for hours, whereas the effects of quiet rest are more transient. Exercise can reduce anxiety even in individuals who are physically limited and frustrated with their ability to perform.

Exercise helps you blow off steam. It's like an anxiety-overflow valve that can bring relief and calm. This is because exercise stimulates the release of endorphins, the soothing chemicals inside you that help relieve pain and anxiety. When done correctly, exercise can also relieve muscle tension, make you less reactive to stress, and help you sleep better. In one study, bicycling was found to be helpful in anxiety reduction, while in another, yoga produced the greatest effect on clear thinking.

Exercising can also make you look better, which in turn can affect your body image and confidence. Overexercising, however, can bring on more anxiety, fatigue, and muscle pain.

■ What Type of Exercise Is Best?

- Martial arts may be best for reducing depression.
- Lifting weights or running can improve confidence.
- Boxing or tennis can help you deal with anger or frustration.
- Team sports may work well if you feel lonely or lack social skills.
- Hiking can enhance your sense of spirituality.
- Swimming or yoga can decrease anxiety.
- Dancing can unblock creative dams and lift your spirits.

■ When You Should Take It Easy Exercising

You should take it easy exercising and consult your health-care practitioner before beginning any exercise program if you . . .

- have a diagnosed heart condition.
- have frequent pains or pressure in the left or mid-chest area, left neck, shoulder, or arm during or right after exercise.
- have had chest pain in the last month.

- tend to lose consciousness or fall due to dizziness.
- feel extremely breathless after mild exercise.
- were advised to take blood-pressure or heart medication by your health-care practitioner.
- have diagnosed bone or joint problems that could be made worse by high-impact exercise.
- have insulin-dependent diabetes or another diagnosed condition that requires special care.
- haven't been physically active or are middle-aged or older and are planning a vigorous exercise program.

▋ Debunking Exercise Myths

Be sure to debunk any myths that may be preventing you from exercising.

Myth 1: Exercising takes too much time. It only takes a few minutes each day to exercise. If you don't have thirty minutes in your schedule for an exercise break, find two fifteen-minute periods or even three ten-minute periods.

Myth 2: Exercising makes me tired. The fact is, the more physically fit you become, the more energy you have.

Myth 3: I have to be athletic to exercise. Most physical activities do not require any special athletic skills. Many of my clients who found school sports difficult discovered several ways to exercise that appealed to them. For example, walking, which is the perfect exercise, requires no special talent, athletic ability, or equipment.

Myth 4: I'm too old to exercise. You can exercise at any age. Individuals age eighty and older have benefited from exercise programs.

Choosing an Exercise That's Right for Your Lifestyle

You don't have to run in a marathon or swim five miles to benefit from exercise. Check the items in the left column that appeal to you, then see which exercise might be best for you.

It's important for me to . . .	So for exercise, I'll try . . .
___increase my self-esteem	dancing, martial arts, or lifting weights
___feel safe	swimming or tai chi
___feel relaxed	ballroom or line dancing, gardening, or walking
___sleep better	walking, biking, dancing, martial arts
___lose weight	jogging, hiking, rowing, cross-country skiing, treadmill, stair climbing
___be flexible	yoga, tai chi, martial arts

▌Why Walking Is a Good Choice

More than 70 million Americans walk for exercise. An advantage of walking is that you don't need any high-tech equipment or to go anywhere special to work out. It's not like being in a class where there's pressure to keep up. When you walk, you go at your own pace.

Having the right shoes can help. When buying walking shoes . . .

- shop later in the day, when your feet are at their largest size.
- look for a shoe with padded insoles, mid-soles, and heel counters. Make sure the sole is firm, thick, and has good traction. The shoe should also be wide enough to accommodate a medium-weight sock.

When walking . . .

- hold your head high as if a gold cord were attached to the top of your head, pulling you up so you walk tall.
- step lightly, landing with your heel first.
- keep your neck and shoulders relaxed and your back flat.
- roll your weight forward across the sole of your foot, gently pushing off with your toes.
- keep your feet pointed straight ahead and your knees slightly bent.
- swing your arms as you walk.

▮ Consider Weight Lifting

The American College of Sports Medicine believes resistance training provides important benefits for individuals of all ages and abilities. They suggest using the following guidelines when lifting free weights:

- Always warm up with stretches prior to your workout.
- Start with 1-pound weights and work up. Consult a specific weight-lifting exercise book, such as *Definition* by Joyce L. Vedral, PhD.
- Breathe throughout your workout; never hold your breath—it could elevate your blood pressure.
- Use smooth, slow, and controlled motions.
- Maintain good posture—working out in front of a mirror can help.
- Only move the body part you're exercising; keep the rest of your body still.
- Complete 8 to 12 repetitions only; if that's too easy, add more weight.

- Rest every other day to let your muscles recover.
- Stop if you feel any sharp or piercing pains.

▌ Use Yoga to Release Anxiety and Tension

The Tension Release exercise in yoga is like an internal massage that can work out the tension from the top of the back, where all the nerve endings meet and where tightness is felt between the shoulder blades.

1. Stand with your back and head in a straight line, feet together, and arms at your sides.
2. Bend your elbows and bring your hands level with your chest.
3. Extend your arms straight out in front.
4. Push your chest out and bring your arms behind the back, bending your elbows and interlocking your fingers while pressing your palms together.
5. Rotate your shoulders forward and up toward your ears.
6. Pull your shoulders down and try to straighten your elbows.
7. Keep your elbows straight and your arms together and raise your arms a short distance, keeping your trunk still.
8. Work over time at getting your arms up to the level of your shoulders.
9. Slowly lower your arms while keeping your hands together and your elbows straight.
10. Let your head relax forward while allowing your elbows to bend and your shoulders to come forward.
11. Bring your arms around to the front.
12. Without bending your knees, let your arms and head droop toward your feet, and work toward touching your toes.

13. After you have mastered steps 1 through 12, clasp your hands behind your back and reach them toward the ceiling.

The Corpse Pose (also called the Sponge, or the Dead Pose) can reduce anxiety once you practice it.

1. Find a comfortable, quiet spot where you won't be disturbed.
2. Loosen your clothes and remove your shoes.
3. Lie on your back with your arms along your sides, palms up, either on a bed or on a carpet or on a pad on the floor.
4. Close your eyes.
5. Let your breathing slowly move toward your center, your abdominal area.
6. Picture life-giving energy from the surrounding atmosphere being drawn in through your feet, filling your entire body with a calming color as you slowly let your body sink into the comfort of your bed (or floor).
7. Continue breathing in the calming color for up to 30 minutes.

▌Tips on Exercising

No matter what kind of exercise you choose, follow these tips:

- Obtain medical supervision prior to exercise if you're over thirty-five years of age, have chest pain when you exert yourself, get short of breath with mild exertion, have pain in your legs when you walk, have swelling in your ankles, or have been told by a doctor that you have heart disease.
- Use proper equipment and clothing when exercising.

- Avoid exercising for 2 hours after a large meal, and don't eat for an hour after exercising.
- Include at least 10 minutes of warm-up and cool-down exercises in your exercise program.
- If you find you can't talk and exercise at the same time, slow down until you can.
- Remember to breathe throughout your workout.
- Stop before you become overtired, even if you're in a class.
- If you exercise outdoors, be careful not to get sunburned or caught in strong winds.
- Shower and change into dry clothes after you finish your cool-down.

■ Overcoming Other Obstacles to Exercise

Attrition in exercise programs is a major problem. If you aren't motivated to exercise, you won't do it. Making exercise part of your lifestyle is an art in itself. Suggestions for making exercise a safe part of your lifestyle include:

1. Start small and keep it fun. Climb stairs instead of taking the elevator; walk short distances instead of driving; plant a garden, or take an evening stroll as a way to work into exercising.
2. Vary exercise regimes to counter boredom; for example, ride a stationery bike one day, lift weights the next, walk the next, and so on.
3. Keep records of daily and weekly progress and include subjective reactions—moods ("I'm starting to like this"), concentration, and sleep-pattern changes—and objective measures—changes in weight, pulse, the way your clothes fit.

4. Post goals, mottos, pictures of your ideal self-affirmations, plus notes of encouragement.

5. Picture yourself being successful in your exercise endeavors: reducing your exercise, feeling good about yourself, looking better and stronger.

6. Reward yourself each time you finish exercising. Congratulate yourself both for working toward exercise goals and for attaining them. For example, after a month in an exercise program, buy a new pair of running shoes, or treat yourself to a movie.

7. Stop exercising, or at least slow down and consult with your health-care practitioner, if any unusual or unexplainable symptoms occur.

8. If you have trouble motivating yourself, work out with an encouraging friend, or join an exercise class, running club, or fitness center. If you spend more time with people dedicated to exercising, you will be too.

9. If you need additional help, don't hesitate to hire a personal trainer or take a class to learn the proper technique.

∎ Be Sure to Warm Up and Cool Down

Whenever you do anything more strenuous than slow walking, make sure to warm up before each exercise session, and to cool down afterward. This will help ensure that you don't strain your muscles or risk injury.

Here's an easy warm-up to try. (You can also use it as your cool-down.) Remember to breathe throughout.

1. Shrug your shoulders 5–10 times, trying to touch your ears with your shoulders.

2. Do the "backstroke" 5–10 times.

3. Turn your head slowly to the left side, come back to center, and turn it slowly to the right side; repeat 5 times.

4. Standing, pull one knee toward your chest, then the other; 5 times each leg. (If balance is a problem, do this one sitting down.)

5. Keeping your feet together, circle your ankles 5 times clockwise and then 5 times counterclockwise.

6. Spread your feet apart at shoulder width and circle your hips 5 times clockwise and then 5 times counterclockwise.

7. Reach up toward the ceiling with one arm and down toward your knee with the other arm; hold and breathe for a count of 5; then do the reverse.

8. Reach up and over your shoulder and pat yourself on the back with one arm and then with the other.

9. Grab your right wrist with your left hand and pull it out straight in front of you; repeat with left wrist and right hand.

10. Stand with your feet 3 feet apart and your fingers laced behind your back, palms up.

11. Grab a belt with both hands and slide it down and up your back 2–3 times.

12. To warm up your hips and legs, sit on the floor with the soles of your feet together. Press your hands on the inside of your knees and hold for 30 seconds, then relax.

13. Stand about a foot away from a door frame or wall. Keeping your body straight, lean against the door frame or wall, bending first your right knee (feel the pull up the back of your left leg) and then the left knee.

▌ How to Exercise at Work

Type the word *exercise* and tape it to your phone to remind you to do one or more of the following exercises every time the phone rings.

1. Sit in your office chair. Every time the phone rings, pull in your stomach muscles and hold for 5 seconds, but keep breathing, then answer the phone. You may get 50 abdominal exercises a day in a busy office.
2. Sit on your desk. Place your hands by your buttocks, pull your stomach muscles tight, and lift your legs out straight. Push down with your hands and slowly raise your buttocks off the desk. Hold for 5 seconds. Repeat at least three times a day.
3. While sitting in a chair, hold on to the arm rests for balance. Slowly straighten the knees, raising the legs as high as possible. Hold for 5 seconds. Repeat at least three times a day.
4. Sit in a chair with your feet spread 18 inches apart. Place your left palm on the inside of your right knee and your right palm on the inside of your left knee. Slowly squeeze your legs together as your resist with your hands. Hold for 5 seconds, breathing deeply. Never hold your breath. Repeat 3 times daily.
5. Every time you get up from your chair, stretch, putting your arms over your head and reaching for the ceiling.

▌ Exercising in Bed

Many people enjoy doing a simple exercise routine before getting out of bed. These exercises must be done slowly and without jerking, and always on a firm mattress. Make sure to breathe throughout the workout.

Lie flat on your back and . . .

1. keep your arms relaxed at your sides. Breathe in and reach with your toes toward the end of the bed. Feel your torso and legs stretch. Exhale. Repeat 5 times. Relax.
2. reach with both arms over your head to touch the headboard or wall and with your feet reach for the end of the bed. Give your whole body a stretch. Return to original position. Repeat 5 times.
3. shrug your shoulders up and back toward the ears as far as possible; add one repetition per week, working up to a total of 10 repetitions.
4. turn your head slowly to the left and then to the right; add 1 turn of your head per week to a maximum of 10 repetitions.
5. hold your arms out in front of you and rotate your wrists clockwise and then counterclockwise, working up to 10 repetitions.
6. clench your fists, holding for several seconds, then extending the fingers, reaching out as far as possible, working up to 10 repetitions.
7. raise your right leg up as far as possible and return it to the bed, keeping the leg as straight as possible without straining your lower back, working up to 10 repetitions.
8. grasp one knee with both hands and bring it toward your chest while slowly moving your head toward that knee, working up to 5 repetitions with each knee.

9. grasp both knees with both hands and slowly pull them toward your chest while slowly moving your head toward your knees, working up to 10 repetitions.

10. bicycle both legs slowly, completing up to 10 circles.

▌Ways to Avoid Injury

- **Build up your level of activity gradually over a few weeks.** Avoid setting your goals too high at first so that you're not tempted to overdo.

- **Listen to your body.** Your body will warn you with pain, light-headedness, or fatigue when you're overdoing. Pay attention to those messages and stop before you injure yourself.

- **Pay attention to the weather conditions.** If you're exercising outside in the cold, wear warm clothes in layers that you can take off and wrap around your waist as you warm up. Wear mittens, gloves, or socks on your hands to protect them. Always wear a hat; up to 40 percent of your body's heat can be lost through your neck and head. In hot climates drink lots of fluids. Wear a plastic water bottle strapped to your waist if it's especially hot and wear light, loose-fitting clothes. Do not wear rubberized or plastic suits, sweatshirts, or sweatpants to try to lose weight; this type of clothing can cause dangerously high body temperatures and result in heat stroke.

- **Caution:** If you have recently undergone surgery or suffer from severe arthritis or osteoporosis or have orthopedic problems, consult with your health-care practitioner prior to exercising.

▮ How Often and For How Long Should You Exercise?

Try to exercise every day. This may sound like a lot now, but soon it will become part of your daily regime. If thirty minutes a day is too much for you, try fifteen minutes twice a day. Purchase a videotape for aerobics, kick boxing, tai chi, weight lifting, yoga, or some other exercise, or tape your favorite exercise show from TV and work out to it.

Remember not to tire yourself out or stress yourself. Easy does it! If you try to do too much, you will become frustrated and may give up on exercise. Plan your workouts so that you don't overdo. Here's how one of my clients planned his exercise session:

> Jed suffered from anxiety attacks and decided to start exercising to reduce his anxiety. He couldn't go farther than his driveway when he started, so he walked down his driveway and back every morning and every evening. Jed slowly worked up to walking to the end of the block, then around the block, then around two blocks. A month later, he was walking two miles a day. By starting small and working up to his exercise goal, Jed felt good about himself and his ability to control anxiety through exercise. You can, too!

▮ Choosing an Exercise Goal That's Right for You

Now you have enough information to choose well, so it's time to pick an exercise goal that's right for you. Below you'll find some goals to choose from. Select at least one and make an agreement with yourself to follow through, or devise your own exercise goal. It's all up to you.

_____ I promise myself I will sign up for a tai chi class and participate in every session.

___I promise myself I will walk twenty minutes a day, starting tomorrow.

___I promise myself I will buy a weight-lifting book and weights and follow the directions.

___I promise myself I will go dancing for at least an hour three times a week.

___I promise myself I will work in my garden for an hour four days a week.

___I promise myself I will buy a treadmill, stair climber, or stationary bicycle and use it three times a week for twenty minutes.

___I promise myself I will turn on the television before work and actively participate in one of the exercise programs.

___I promise I will sign up for a yoga class and participate at least once a week.

___I promise I will join a health club or sign up for an exercise class and participate at least three times a week.

___I promise myself I will: _____.

▌ Summary

1. Use exercise to reduce anxiety and panic attacks.
2. Find the best way to exercise for you.
3. Make sure you know if you should be taking it easy exercising.
4. Debunk any exercise myths you hold.
5. Learn ways to motivate yourself to exercise.
6. To avoid injury, be sure to always warm up before exercising, and cool down after you finish.

9

Other Anxiety-Reducing and Healing Measures

Relaxation promotes production of the chemical norepinephrine in the body. Low levels of this neurotransmitter can result in depression, so to feel better, participate in activities that foster relaxation.

There are many self-care and healing measures you can use to reduce your anxiety. Unlike medications, most have few or no harmful side effects. Whichever ones you choose, remember that if you want to overcome the fears or needs beneath your anxiety, you must face them. Stop waiting for circumstances to be just right before you act. Take small steps toward reducing your anxiety. As the saying goes, nothing ventured, nothing gained. If your anxiety is still bothering you as you read this, it's time to make a change and try something new.

As you start to see accomplishments from trying one or more of the procedures in this chapter, you'll feel new strength and improved self-esteem. Remember to acknowledge the positive things in your life. Even when you're anxious, make a real effort to remember some past positive experiences instead of focusing on the negative ones. Avoid catastrophic thinking. Ask yourself, "What is the worst thing that could happen in this situation?" You'll usually find the outcome is something you can survive, even though it might not be pleasant. Once you face the unpleasant situation, rather than try to hide from it, your self-esteem will soar. You'll be proud of yourself for taking control and conquering your fears.

Aim to stay focused. Much of your anxiety is the result of projecting yourself into future situations. Stay in the present, the here and now. That's the only thing you can control, anyway.

Take one step at a time and give yourself permission to retry an approach. You can go back and redo steps of the approach as many times as you need to so that you're comfortable and satisfied with the outcome.

In this chapter you'll discover the anxiety-reducing and healing measures I've found most useful and effective, both personally and professionally. They're listed alphabetically for easy reference. I suggest you read through all of them before deciding which one(s) to try first. Keep in mind that combining measures is often more powerful. For example, imagery, progressive relaxation, and self-hypnosis work well together.

▌ Accepting Your Anxiety

Often when you try to control your anxiety or pretend it's not there, your anxiety builds. Claim it. Let go of your need to control and try anxiety-management strategies instead. Be patient with yourself and take it one day at a time. Chart your progress by keeping track of your moments of anxiety and when they occur. Once you do that, you've already started to gain a sense of real control because you now have enough information to do something about it.

▪ Act As If

Role-playing practice can help you act the way you want in upcoming anxiety-provoking situations. Find a supportive partner and practice acting the way you wish you could be. You may surprise yourself and find something within that you never knew you had. Begin with the idea that you'll only make small changes, then try out your idea and pay attention to what happened when you tried to act differently. Remember, you don't have to perform perfectly, you're only practicing. Be brave and see what happens.

Ted wanted to ask Doris to marry him, but he was anxious about proposing, fearing she might reject him. He tried to tell himself she'd agree to his proposal, but it didn't work and he still worried. Practicing role-playing with his counselor, Ted found he was able to stay calm even when his counselor didn't react positively to his proposal. They practiced the scene several times in several different ways until Ted felt confidant he could handle Doris's response, no matter what it was.

▪ Accomplishment List

Before you end your day, write down the five most important things you want to accomplish the next day. Be sure to be specific. Number each in order of its importance. The next day, start working on your number-one priority. Try to complete as many as you can that day, but don't worry if you can't finish them all, because you will always be working on what is number one in importance to you. If you find your top priority seems too overwhelming, break it down into manageable steps, two or more high-priority goals to work on. Give yourself a pat on the back each time you accomplish one of your priorities.

▌Acupressure

You can use your fingers to release anxiety. Acupressure is the use of the fingertips on specific body points to release blocked energy. One of the simplest acupressure holds that can reduce anxiety is to rub the webbing between your thumb and index finger.

To prepare yourself to use light-touch acupressure, place the three middle fingers of your right or left hand on the outer aspect of your other forearm. Let your finger pads rest lightly on your other arm. Use enough pressure so you can begin to feel a pulsation coming from the fingertips. Balance the pulsation in all three fingers so that they match and are strong and even. This is the effect you will strive for in each of the areas of your body listed below.

1. To the right and left of the spinal cord where your neck meets your shoulder.
2. Above your little finger at the point where your hand meets your wrist.
3. Just below the collarbone, about in the middle, at a point that lines up with your ears.
4. At the bottom of the middle of your ribs on both sides of your body.
5. In the middle of the point where your legs attach to your body.
6. At the insides of both knees.
7. At the inside of both heels, in a line with your big toes.
8. At the bottom of your big toes.

Calm can be restored by massaging points on the body as follows:

1. In the middle of the spinal column, halfway down the shoulder blades.

2. On either side of the ninth thoracic vertebra, about the level of the nipples.

3. On the front of the body on the sternum.

4. Just below the navel.

5. Between the diaphragm and navel.

■ Acupuncture

Acupuncture involves the insertion of stainless-steel needles at precise anatomic locations. The needles may be stimulated by moxibustion (the burning of the herb *Artemisia vulgaris)* and cupping, a suctioning of the skin through the application of small jars in which a vacuum is created. Magnets of various sizes and shapes may also be used. Your insurance company may even pay for it. Acupuncture practitioners use pulse or tongue diagnosis, and talk about your *qi*, or energy, and whether substances are Yin or Yang.

Sam suffered from frequent anxiety attacks that included rapid heartbeat, difficulty sleeping through the night, restlessness, and dry mouth. He tried psychotherapy but it wasn't helping. A friend told Sam about the benefits of acupuncture and Sam tried it. He slept deeply during the first treatment. Eight treatments later, Sam reported that his psychotherapy was now going well and he was sleeping through the night.

If you're chronically anxious, you may be too tense to relax, let alone sleep well. Acupuncture can often bring on a deep state of relaxation. Acupuncture can also help you relax enough to bring to the forefront emotional issues that are holding you back. If you decide to have acupuncture, carefully observe (and have someone else record) your moods, dreams, or unusual mental states that can occur for several days after a treatment.

■ Affirmations

Affirmations are positive thoughts you choose to immerse your consciousness in to produce a desired effect.

We all carry on negative dialogues with ourselves. Called "self-talk" by Dr. Albert Ellis, author of *A Guide to Rational Living*, much of this is left over from earlier family experiences. Affirmations provide positive messages to counteract negative messages we have received and may be inflicting on ourselves.

Louise Hay, guru of affirmations, suggests in *Heal Your Body* that anxiety is due to not trusting the flow and the process of life. She suggests repeating, "I love and approve of myself and I trust the process of life. I am safe."

There are other affirmations that may also be of help to you. Choose from the list of affirmations below or devise your own positive statements. Just make sure you either say or write them twenty times a day for at least a week. It is also suggested that you write your affirmations on three-by-five cards and place them on your bathroom mirror, on your desk, in your bag or briefcase, and any places that you visit frequently.

Some affirmations to choose from include:

- I am becoming more and more relaxed.
- I can relax and breathe calmly.
- Whenever I feel anxious, I'll fill my body with a peaceful light (color, sound, or word).
- I am responsible for making myself feel good.
- I decide for myself.
- I can see the positive in any situation.
- I believe in myself.
- I decide and then act.

- It's getting easier and easier to exercise (to eat in ways that reduce my anxiety, to change my work environment, to change my home environment).

Affirmations Especially for Panic

- I can do abdominal breathing and say "Stop!" to all scary thoughts, and my anxiety will subside in a few minutes.
- If I get negative criticism at work, I can find out what I need to change in my behavior and make a plan.
- If I lose my job, I'll look for something part-time and use my savings until I find what I want to do that is less stressful.
- If I fall due to shaky legs, I can sit there for a few minutes until my anxiety subsides; even if I feel embarrassed, I can handle it.
- Even if my heart beats fast, the doctor said I have a healthy heart that can handle a few minutes of heavy beating.
- I'm not going to faint from anxiety; fainting is due to low blood pressure, and anxiety raises my blood pressure.
- Even if I feel spacey or not myself, I know it will pass once I relax and take a few abdominal breaths.
- Even if I do have a heart condition, I can change my diet, exercise and stress patterns, and learn to strengthen my heart.
- Anxiety is making it seem like I can't breathe, but if I relax my diaphragm with slow, easy breaths, the feeling will go away.
- Even if I get anxious when I have to confront someone about something, I can stay focused. Even if that person gets angry, I can do abdominal breathing and picture myself protected behind a plastic shield that doesn't let in any negative effects.

- I may feel scared, but I've never acted crazy; anxiety never turns into crazy action.
- If I feel hot or cold, I can relax because I know it's just stress hormones doing it, and my temperature will go back to normal in a few minutes.
- Even if someone does steal my money, I can cope and run for help.
- There's no need for me to panic; I'll just do controlled breathing, say "peace" over and over to myself, and wait it out for a few minutes until my anxiety drops.

Affirmations Especially for Phobias and Fears

- High-rises have safety glass that's thick and there's no way I can fall through a sealed, thick glass window; the worst that could happen is I could trip and then get my balance back.
- My body has a good immune system and if I wash my hands after touching other people, I will be safe.
- Although I feel very anxious when I get up high, I can work up to being up high, and focus on counting my breaths to stay calm.
- Although I may feel anxious around dogs (or cats, snakes, or insects), if I stay calm and focus on counting my breaths and picturing myself and the creature remaining calm, the other creature will stay calmer because I will be putting out less adrenaline.
- Although I may feel anxious when I leave home, I can focus on counting my breaths and slowly work up to being outside and feeling calm.
- Although I may feel anxious when I go shopping (to the dentist, the doctor, the beautician) I can focus on counting my breaths, picture myself looking peaceful, and slowly work up to being in a store (at the dentist, the doctor, the beautician) and feeling calm.

- Although I may feel anxious about driving (taking public transportation, flying, etc.), I can focus on counting my breaths, picture myself staying calm, and slowly work up to traveling and staying calm.
- Although I may feel anxious when I go through tunnels (under bridges, up elevators, on escalators), I can slowly work up to being in them (under them, riding on them), count my breaths, and picture myself looking calm, and I will stay calm.
- Although I may feel anxious being alone (in the dark, or when it thunders, or when there is lightening), I can count my breaths and picture myself staying calm, and I will.

Affirmations Especially for Intrusive Thoughts and Ritualistic Actions

- Even though I believe I may hurt or harm a close relative, I can stay calm by counting my breaths and picturing myself getting along with the person.
- Even though I've checked, and even though I still believe I have to go back and lock my door (turn off an appliance), I know it's just anxiety and I can stay calm by counting my breaths and picturing the door locked (appliance off).
- Even though I know I'm 99.99 percent safe from a catastrophe occurring, I still believe I'm not safe, but I know it's just anxiety and I can stay calm by counting my breaths and picturing my surroundings peaceful and calm.

Affirmations Especially for Post-Traumatic Stress

- Even though I know it is just my anxiety triggering a replay of past experiences, I know I can stay calm if I count my breaths and picture myself calm and peaceful.
- Even though I know it is just my anxiety triggering a replay, I know I can stay calm if I write in my journal, draw

pictures that are calming and peaceful, or listen to my relaxation tape.

- Even though thoughts and images of my trauma sometime come back, I can say "Stop" to end them, or if that doesn't work I can snap the rubber band on my wrist and they will disappear.

- If a flood of traumatic memories comes back, I can swim, walk, or play tennis to reduce my tension and anxiety.

- If I feel dead inside or in a faraway world, I can bring myself back to reality by taking a bath or shower, touching a safe object (such as a stuffed animal), stretching and doing sit-ups, writing in my journal, or talking to a supportive person.

- If I start feeling jittery and anxious, I can deep-breathe or picture myself in a safe, calm place, go to my assertiveness class, or stop ingesting so much sugar and caffeine.

- I forgive myself and stop blaming myself for whatever happened.

When Affirmations Don't Come Easily

You may be able to use affirmations right away and find them useful. Or you may be like Julie and need to take a different approach.

Julie, a twenty-one-year-old college student, was having difficulty following through with her exercise regime to control her anxiety. She had heard about affirmations and asked me how to use them. I proceeded to help her find an appropriate affirmation to use. At first it seemed she was ready to develop an affirmation to exercise, but as we talked it became clear she wasn't ready to take responsibility for exercising. That's when we phrased the following affirmation: "I, Julie, am finding it easier and easier to accept the idea of exercising to relieve my anxiety."

The first few weeks Julie repeated the affirmation she didn't seem to believe what she was saying. By the second week she said, "You know, maybe exercising will help." Julie continued saying her affirmation and carried the written form of it with her on a three-by-five card wherever she went. The following week, Julie said she had mastered the affirmation and was ready to develop an affirmation about exercising. She chose the following affirmation: "It's getting easier and easier to exercise every day." By the next week, she had enrolled in a yoga class and was taking line-dancing lessons.

■ Alexander Method

The Alexander Technique is a way to help you let go of anxiety and tension through mind/body awareness. The most important word here is *let*. The theory is that if you deliberately try to move a neck that's stiff from anxiety or force anxiety-paralyzed legs to move, it won't work. Instead, think of freeing your neck. That way, your mind sends a message to your neck muscles to let go of tension.

Try the application that follows to see if this method may be beneficial for you.

1. Lie on a carpeted floor or mat.
2. Place enough books under your head to make sure your head doesn't press back and down.
3. Bend your knees up and keep your feet flat on the floor; place your hands on your rib cage.
4. Merely think or say the following directions to yourself as you lie still, without trying to make them happen:
   Let my neck be free to let my head go forward and up . . .
   to let my torso lengthen and widen . . .
   to let my legs release from my torso . . .
   and let my shoulders widen.

▪ Autogenics

Autogenic Training (AT) is a systematic program you can use to relax and reduce your anxiety. You use verbal commands to effectively reduce your anxiety. AT was developed by Oskar Vogt, a famous brain physiologist in the nineteenth century. He taught individuals to put themselves into a trance to reduce tension and fatigue. The goal of AT is to normalize the physical, mental, and emotional processes that can become unbalanced by anxiety. Johannes H. Schultz, a Berlin psychiatrist, found that you can create a state very much like an hypnotic trance just by thinking of heaviness and warmth in your extremities.

AT has proven to be most effective with generalized anxiety, but it can also increase your resistance to anxiety and reduce or eliminate sleeping disorders. At least one study found that autogenic training provided relief for the majority of participants suffering from panic. AT should not be used with children under age five, or with anyone suffering from a severe mental or emotional disorder. Check with your health-care practitioner if you have a chronic disease such as diabetes, or heart conditions or high blood pressure. If you feel very anxious or restless while practicing AT or experience disquieting side effects, discontinue AT or use it under the supervision of a professional AT instructor.

Take from four to ten months to master all six exercises, using one- and half-minute sessions five to eight times a day. As you become more comfortable with AT, gradually increase the length of sessions to thirty or forty minutes twice a day. Just let what happens happen and don't try to analyze it.

There are three AT positions:

1. Sitting in an armchair that supports your head, back, and extremities comfortably.

2. Sitting on a stool and stooping over with your arms resting on your thighs, your hands draped between your knees.

3. Lying down with your head supported on a pillow, your legs about eight inches apart, your toes pointed slightly outward, and your arms resting comfortably at your sides without touching them.

Adjust the AT program to your own pace. Be patient and don't move too fast; make sure you've mastered one exercise before moving on to the next one. If you have trouble achieving a sense of heaviness, picture heaviness, weights weighing you down, gently sinking, or whatever works for you. If you have difficulty experiencing a feeling of warmth, picture your arm lying on a warm heating pad or imagine being in a nice warm shower or bath, or sitting outside in the sunshine. If you have difficulty becoming aware of your heartbeat, hold your hand over your heart.

Weeks one to three focus on heaviness. Weeks four to seven focus on warmth. Week eight focuses on heartbeat, week nine on breathing, week ten on your solar plexus (skip this one if you have ulcers, diabetes, or any bleeding in your abdominal organs), week eleven focuses on your forehead, and week twelve focuses on individualized themes.

Week 1: Start with your right arm and repeat each statement four times. (If you're left-handed, start with your left.)
My right arm is heavy.
My left arm is heavy.
Both of my arms are heavy.

Week 2: Repeat the following statements for 3 minutes, four to seven times a day.
My right arm is heavy.
My left arm is heavy.

Both of my arms are heavy.
My right leg is heavy.
My left leg is heavy.
Both my legs are heavy.
My arms and legs are heavy.

Week 3: Repeat the following statements for three minutes, four to seven times a day.
My right arm is heavy.
Both of my arms are heavy.
Both of my legs are heavy.
My arms and legs are heavy.

Week 4: Repeat the following statements for 5 minutes, four to seven times a day.
My right arm is heavy.
My arms and legs are heavy.
My right arm is warm.
My left arm is warm.
Both of my arms are warm.

Week 5: Repeat the following statements for 8 minutes, three to six times a day.
My right arm is heavy.
My arms and legs are heavy.
My right arm is warm.
My left arm is warm.
My right leg is warm.
Both of my legs are warm.
My arms and legs are warm.

Week 6: Repeat the following statements for 10–15 minutes, three to six times a day.

My right arm is heavy.
My arms and legs are heavy.
Both of my arms are warm.
Both of my legs are warm.
My arms and legs are warm.
My arms and legs are heavy and warm.

Week 7: Repeat the following for 10–20 minutes, three to six times a day.
My right arm is heavy.
My arms and legs are heavy.
My arms and legs are warm.
My arms and legs are heavy and warm.

Week 8: Say aloud the following statements for 10–20 minutes, three to six times a day. (If you experience any distress with this one, stop it and try again in week 11.)
My right arm is heavy.
My arms and legs are heavy and warm.
My heartbeat is calm and regular.

Week 9: Say aloud the following statements for 10–20 minutes, three to six times a day.
My right arm is heavy and warm.
My arms and legs are heavy and warm.
My heartbeat is calm and regular.
It breathes me.

Week 10: Say aloud the following statements for 10–20 minutes, three to six times a day.
My right arm is heavy and warm.
My arms and legs are heavy and warm.
My heartbeat is calm and regular.

It breathes me.

My solar plexus is warm.

Week 11: Say aloud the following statements while lying on your back for 10–20 minutes, three to six times a day.

My right arm is heavy and warm.

My arms and legs are heavy and warm.

My heartbeat is calm and regular.

It breathes me.

My solar plexus is warm.

My forehead is cool.

Week 12: Say one or more of the following statements for 10–20 minutes, three to six times a day.

My mind is quiet.

I feel serene and still.

I am at ease.

I picture and experience myself as relaxed and comfortable.

I feel quiet and serene.

I feel an inward quietness.

■ Breathing Awareness

Breathing is essential for life. If you're breathing in the upper part of your chest, not allowing sufficient blood to oxygenate the lungs, brain, and other tissues, you may be adding to your anxiety.

When anxious, you are probably restricting your breathing even more, increasing muscular tension, anxiety, and irritability. Have you noticed how when you feel anxious, you tend to halt your breathing? When you start to feel anxious, deep breathing can help relax you. But there is a specific way to breathe to obtain anxiety reduction.

Relaxing breathing is deep and comes from the diaphragm or abdomen. Tense breathing occurs in the upper chest and is fast and shallow.

Become aware of how you breathe by:

1. sitting comfortably in a relaxed position;
2. closing your eyes and placing your hands over your navel; then,
3. without making any effort to change, noticing whether your stomach is expanding out or flattening as you exhale.

To achieve abdominal breathing, begin finding a quiet environment where you won't be disturbed. As you reduce noise and other demands on you, your mind will turn inward. Begin to notice the rhythmic rise and fall of your chest. As you focus on your breathing, you will naturally begin to breathe more slowly and deeply and your body will shift into a more relaxed mode. Gently suggest to your body that your breathing will move lower in your body, toward your middle, toward your navel.

Harvard psychologist Dr. Joan Borysenko, author of *Minding the Body, Mending the Mind,* is one of many mental-health professionals who believes that breathing effectively is a great way to break a cycle of anxiety. When you keep your mind and body busy with breathing, anxiety disappears.

Alternate Nostril Breathing

One way to calm the mind and reduce anxiety is through alternate nostril breathing. This type of breathing, as well as others, can rapidly reduce blood pressure. Use the directions that follow:

1. Sit in a comfortable chair or lie down.
2. Close your left nostril with the fourth and fifth fingers of your right hand and inhale deeply and slowly through your right nostril.

3. Hold for several seconds, then close your right nostril with your thumb, open your left nostril, and exhale through it.
4. Repeat steps 2 and 3 (above) five times each; over time, add one more alternate nostril breath a day.

Breathing and Imagery

Breathing can be combined with imagery to reduce anxiety.

1. Find a comfortable place and either sit or lie down.
2. Place your hands on your abdomen.
3. When you inhale, picture relaxing energy flowing through you, filling you up.
4. When you exhale, picture yourself releasing whatever it's time to let go of.

Breathing Retraining

Rapid, shallow breathing (hyperventilation) can bring on panic, heart palpitations, and other symptoms associated with fearful situations. In one study, individuals trained to breathe normally while being exposed to threatening environments showed a marked decrease in their fear of being in open or strange areas and of leaving the house (agoraphobia).

Based on a combined analysis of twenty-eight published studies, researchers concluded that relaxation training and controlled exposure to panic-inducing situations are two very effective psychological techniques. Breathing retraining uses these two approaches to help you prevent panic attacks.

To retrain your breathing, you must learn to feel relaxed while doing abdominal breathing and then picture upsetting situations. This builds up a history of breathing calmly while picturing an upsetting situation (your brain doesn't know the difference between imagining an upsetting situation and experiencing one) that you can call upon and use during real-life events.

Follow the directions given below to retrain your breathing:

1. Lie on your back on a carpet or bed in a quiet spot where you won't be interrupted.
2. Place your hands on your abdomen and gently suggest to your breathing that it move toward the center of your body. Notice how your hands begin to move out with your abdomen as you inhale and come back as you exhale.
3. Continue breathing in this manner as you begin to feel more comfortable.
4. Begin to think about a situation that is of minor concern to you. Stop thinking about that situation if you start to feel anxious and return to abdominal breathing until you feel comfortable again.
5. Return to thinking about the chosen situation until you can picture yourself staying calm and relaxed through the whole situation. You can return to abdominal breathing anytime you wish.
6. Now choose a situation of a little more concern to you and repeat steps 4 and 5.
7. Keep choosing situations that result in slightly more anxiety for you and repeat steps 4 and 5 until you feel comfortable in each situation.

Identifying Overbreathing

When you're anxious, you breathe more rapidly and shallowly. You may even have an ongoing tendency to overbreathe. This kind of breathing sets you up for hyperventilation. Look for the following signs:

- irregular breaths
- gasping for breath
- shallow breathing in the upper chest

- sighing
- yawning
- frequent clearing of the throat
- heavy breathing

Although hyperventilation is harmless, it can give you the impression you don't have enough air to breathe, that you're smothering or breathless. If you're a woman, you may have been taught to hold your stomach in and your chest up. This can lead to shallow breathing and hyperventilation.

There are four things you can do to stop hyperventilation:

1. Breathe in and out of a paper bag.
2. Hold your breath a few times in a row.
3. Participate in vigorous exercise such as running up and down stairs, do aerobics in place, or walk briskly.
4. Learn abdominal breathing. (See Breathing Retraining, above.)

▮ Chromotherapy

Chromotherapy is the use of color to heal. It has been practiced since ancient times in early Greece, China, and India. The theory behind chromotherapy is that colors of light in the visible spectrum are lower "octaves" of higher vibrational energies that affect the chakras, or energy centers, of the body. The crown chakra, located at the top of the head, is the focus of treatment in anxiety. In this case, the color to be used is violet. You can wear violet clothes, buy swatches (one foot by one foot) of violet cotton cloth and place them on painful areas, or visualize breathing in the color violet. Use the directions that follow for color breathing:

1. Sit in a comfortable position with your eyes closed.
2. Breathe, letting your breathing slowly move toward your center, your abdomen.
3. As you inhale, see and feel the color violet. Visualize violet color filling up your entire body.
4. Imagine this colored breath healing and balancing whatever is needed by your body at this time.
5. Continue this process for 10 minutes, then open your eyes and enjoy the sensation of calm.

Depending on the issues you're facing, you can also use other colors, specifically:

- Indigo if you have obsessions
- Blue to relax and cool your body
- Green to awaken your hope, faith, and friendliness
- Peach to reduce emotional paralysis
- Gold to provide a feeling of protection
- Brown to calm and stabilize overexcited states

■ Coping Skills

Coping-skills training includes a combination of progressive relaxation and stress-coping self-statements that are used to replace the defeatist self-talk called forth in stressful situations. You can rehearse coping-skills procedures in your imagination to prepare for real-life events that raise your level of anxiety.

This rehearsal is important, because according to Dr. Aaron Beck, author of *Cognitive Therapy of Anxiety and Phobic Disorders,* we all respond to situations with a tendency to think and react in a certain way. In the cognitive therapy approach, the thought that precedes the feeling is changed to elicit more positive emotion. If you tend to be depressed, you will interpret a splash of water from a passing car during a rainstorm as convincing proof that you are a failure, there is no need in proceeding any further with the day, and you might as well go back home to bed and pull the covers over your head.

If you suffer from anxiety, you will probably interpret situations like the water splash as a personal danger or threat. If you have a tendency to obsess, you're probably most likely to interpret the rain splash as evidence of threat of contamination. If you have social anxiety, you may start to sweat, flush, and shake, the very things you're anxious about doing and having other people observe. If you tend to have panic attacks, you may interpret a speeding-up of your heart after being splashed as a sign of a heart attack that requires immediate medical attention.

Unfortunately, when you interpret an event as a threat, the tendency is to seek safety and avoid anxiety-provoking situations, but this only increases your anxiety because you're apt to tell yourself, "See, this was a near miss. In the future I mustn't be around any of these situations that make me anxious." As a result, you are constantly anxious, not wanting to be anywhere near the feared situation. In reality, it is only by confronting the feared situation and seeing that you can survive that you will reduce your anxiety and learn to live with much less fear.

You can see how anxiety can be evoked just by your attitude. Do you enter situations thinking you're going to be anxious and uncomfortable? With this kind of mindset you are poised to feel anxious. That's why coping skills are so important. They can help you enter a situation believing in yourself and your ability to stay calm.

Hint: If you break your preparation for an upcoming situation into four parts, you will have more success.

The first task is to prepare: take a deep breath and begin to focus on the task. Second: interrupt any negative thoughts that come into your mind and tell yourself you can stay calm and confident. Third: pay attention to your feelings. When they start to build, begin to use positive statements to talk yourself through the situation, comments such as "I can do this. I have confidence in my ability." And, fourth: learn to cope with feelings as they start to build by using positive comments to yourself such as "I'm anxious, but I can handle it. I've handled it before." Once the situation is over, reward yourself for what you've accomplished. Recognize any small movement toward your goal to remain calm.

Coping thoughts can be divided into statements used for the different stages in dealing with an anxiety-provoking situation: preparation, the situation, and reinforcing success. Here are some examples.

Preparatory Stage
Use the statements that follow prior to the anxiety-provoking situation.

- I can handle this.
- There's nothing to worry about.
- I'll jump in and be all right.
- It will be easier once I get started.
- Soon this will be over.

The Situation
Use these statements during the anxiety-provoking situation.

- I will not allow this situation to upset me.
- Take a deep breath and relax.
- I can take it step by step.
- I can do this; I'm handling it now.
- I can keep my mind on the task at hand.
- It doesn't matter what others think; I will do it.
- Deep breathing really works.

Reinforcing Success

Once the situation is over, use these statements to reward yourself and increase the chances you'll stay calm in future situations.

- Situations don't have to overwhelm me anymore.
- I did it!
- I did well.
- I'm going to tell_____(name of person) about my success.
- By not thinking about being anxious, I wasn't anxious.

These procedures have been shown effective for reducing general anxiety, as well as for anxiety due to interviews, public speaking, and tests. They also can help with phobias, especially fear of heights. Follow the guidelines below.

1. Find a quiet spot where you won't be interrupted and think of an anxiety-provoking situation.
2. Choose several coping thoughts or statements (see above) for each stage of an anxiety-provoking situation, and write them on three-by-five cards. Use these statements when you practice, and carry them with you to use in upsetting situations.
3. Get your body relaxed by consciously relaxing your body or listening to a relaxation tape. (See Progressive Relaxation.)
4. Picture yourself in the anxiety-provoking situation, or if you can't relax enough that way, picture yourself during the period prior to the anxiety-provoking situation. Say or think your coping-skills statements, using the ones relevant to the stage you're in.

5. Work back and forth between picturing the situation, saying your coping-skills statements, and relaxing your body until you complete the whole situation in a relaxed state.

■ Focus on the Now

Focusing on the past or future can increase your anxiety. Stay focused on the present, and what is actually happening, not with your interpretation of what you think is happening. Focus on the outcome of what you plan to do, not on your fears or anxiety. When you let your emotions control you, the intensity of the moment can limit your options. Decide what your goal is and focus on that.

Phoebe felt anxious in public situations. She worried constantly about what other people thought of her. This created intense anxiety for her. When Phoebe's boss told her she was going to have to speak to the employees about a new procedure, she panicked. Phoebe asked me to help her deal with this new and frightening request. I asked her to focus on just one or two of the people in the audience whom she knew and trusted. I asked her to imagine herself talking to the large group, but picture herself having eye contact with just a few people in the audience. She reported that her anxiety lessened as she pictured her friends smiling and nodding at her as she spoke. I suggested she ask her friends to sit throughout the audience, identify themselves to her before she began to speak, and to smile and nod at her throughout her presentation. Phoebe reported to me after the presentation and told me the approach we'd agreed on had worked well.

❚ Imagery

You already have had experiences with self-generated images in dreams, daydreams, and fantasies. Most children have a well-developed sense of imaging. As they grow older, their skills may become dormant as the logical, rational (left) side of their brain is used in schoolwork and linear thought processes.

Imagery is a powerful tool for reducing anxiety. The power of this approach is derived from its right-brain source. Your right brain, which controls the left side of your body, is primarily responsible for orientation in space, body image, artistic endeavor, and recognition of faces. The right side of your brain deals with visual, holistic, intuitive, nonlinear thought. Imagery allows direct access to your subconscious and the autonomic-nervous-system functions, bypassing the left brain and its tendency to solve problem through logical reasoning. It is often logical processing that can lead to the repetitive worrying that increases anxiety. Imagery can cut through rumination to the essential core of issues and lead to effective problem solving, decreased anxiety, and increased self-confidence. Your mind doesn't differentiate between an image of a situation and the actual experience of being in the situation, so a great deal of learning can occur during imagery. Once you picture yourself in an anxiety-provoking situation, you increase your ability to remain calm and relaxed in a similar real-life situation in the future.

Sarah, a recent college graduate, told me she was anxious about asking her boss for a raise. I suggested she try imagery to prepare for the confrontation. Sarah agreed to give it a try. I played a relaxation tape for her and asked her to signal me with her index finger when she felt relaxed. When she signaled me, I asked her to imagine herself as the director of a movie starring herself, with her boss as the supporting actor. I asked her to picture herself going to her boss's office and to continue with the scene until she felt anxious, and then to signal me by raising her index finger. We worked back and forth like this until Sarah opened her eyes and exclaimed, "I got through the whole situation without feeling anxious." I then asked her to continue practicing this process at home and advised her she would notice that it became easier and easier to get through the scene, and as that happened, it would be even easier to talk to her boss about a raise.

You can use this kind of imagery process yourself to reduce your anxiety about upcoming situations. Use the following guidelines to practice:

1. Decide on an upcoming situation for practice. Choose a situation you are anxious about, one whose outcome you worry about or need practice handling in a calm manner.
2. Assume a comfortable position in a place where you won't be interrupted, with your body relaxed and your eyes closed.
3. If you have difficulty relaxing, use a relaxation tape, either one you purchased or one you made yourself. (See Progressive Relaxation.)
4. Imagine yourself as the director of a movie that you are going to run in your mind's eye. As director, you can start or stop the movie at any point where discomfort occurs.
5. Begin the movie, imagining everything about the situation, from what is said, what you feel, to what the other persons in the situation say and do. When you notice yourself becoming uncomfortable, stop the movie in your mind and return to focusing on relaxing your body.

When you're relaxed again, begin the movie at the spot a little before you felt anxious. Continue the movie until you feel uncomfortable or displeased with what occurs, and return to relaxing. Work back and forth between the movie in your mind and relaxing until you can complete the whole situation while remaining relaxed.

You can also use imagery to decrease painful or negative feelings. Follow the directions below to use imagery in this manner.

1. Use a relaxation tape or picture yourself in a quiet, peaceful place to relax your body.
2. Scan your body and find the areas where your anxiety resides.
3. Think of a container for your anxiety and picture it vividly.
4. Place all of your anxiety in the container and put a tight lid on it and lock it tightly.
5. Place the locked container in a place where it can no longer influence you.

When you encounter difficulty with completing this exercise, it may be because you aren't ready to give up your anxiety. If this is the case with you, check out the Affirmations section (above) for ways to help you get ready to give up your anxiety.

You can also use imagery during an anxiety attack. Practice at home when you are in a safe, relatively nonthreatening environment. Once you learn the technique, you can use it at work, at school, or anywhere you experience anxiety.

1. Close your eyes and breathe out three times. See yourself at the seashore. The sky is clear, the breeze is warm and comforting on you. See and feel your anxiety as a rock. Watch the water and wind erode this rock, washing and blowing it away. Know that when the rock is gone, your anxiety will also be gone. When that happens, open your eyes and enjoy the relaxed feeling.

2. Close your eyes and breathe out three times. See yourself being calm, like the surface of a calm lake. When you feel that all anxiety has passed, open your eyes.

■ Immersion

When you are immersed in a pleasurable event, anxiety will recede. Take a minute or two to . . .

- smell a flower
- appreciate a sunrise
- watch the sun set
- enjoy the warmth of the sun on your skin
- enjoy a bite of food or another simple but enjoyable experience

Really let yourself enjoy the experience and immerse yourself in it, forgetting everything else. Here are some more positive experiences to immerse yourself in:

- Listen to a cassette or CD of soothing music.
- Wear clothes that make you feel good.
- Buy a plant for your work desk.
- Take a warm bath or sauna.

Take a few minutes right now to write down activities you like to do that help relax you. Explore whether you like physical, social, emotional, creative, or intellectual activities, and when and where you like to do the activity.

▌Inner-Directed Movement

It may seem silly to suggest that something as simple as yawning could reduce anxiety, improve your well-being, and even revolutionize the way you feel about yourself, but inner-directed movement can do just that. Try the exercise that follows and see if inner-directed movement helps reduce your anxiety.

1. Set aside 10–20 minutes and wear clothes suitable for easy movement.
2. Play some music that is flowing but without a strong beat.
3. Stand in a quiet place, somewhere you won't be disturbed.
4. Let your head drop back, open your mouth, and pretend to yawn. A natural yawn may start, and if it does, let it take over. Allow yourself a luxurious yawn and continue to yawn as long and as many times as you want, letting your arms and body get involved. Allow whatever sounds you wish to make to come out. Groaning or moaning may work better for you. Experiment and see. Think of this as playtime.

▌Journaling

Recording your thoughts and feelings is a great way to catch the negative things you think and say about yourself and others. Journaling, or journal writing, is a way to establish a permanent record of your thoughts, feelings, and situations that evoke anxiety. Journal writing has been shown to be more effective for clients with PTSD than cognitive therapy. Writing about emotions is especially useful in helping heal PTSD, but it can also be effective for other sources of anxiety.

When you journal, make an entry when you identify a painful

thought. First comes the thought, and then the feeling, so if you can identify thoughts that lead to anxiety, you will be more ready to catch them, to say "cancel that thought" or perform "thought stopping" (see below).

You may wish to use the format Sarah used when she wrote about thoughts that bothered her.

Situation	Automatic Thoughts	Feelings
Saturday night . . . at a party with my husband at his boss's house	"I'm going to blow this for him."	anxiety, panic
Monday morning . . . my boss asks me to write a report	"I'll never be able to do this."	anxiety
Have to work a double shift . . . can't meet husband for dinner	"Chad's going to have a fit."	anxiety

■ Massage

Getting a massage from a partner, friend, or massage therapist can be an excellent way to reduce your anxiety. There are also specific points you can massage, depending on your symptoms.

For anxiety: massage the webbing between your thumbs and index fingers.

For heart fluttering and dizziness: massage with firm pressure for just ten to twenty seconds at the following points:

- In the depression on the right side of your neck below the bone that goes along the back of your head.
- On a diagonal across the left arm where it meets the shoulder.

- Both thighs, on the inner and outer aspects.
- On the middle back of the right lower leg.

▌ Meditation

Meditation is the process of focusing your attention on one thing at a time, uncritically and totally. You can repeat a syllable, word, a group of words, aloud or silently. This is called *mantra meditation*. You can count your breaths aloud or silently. This is called *breath-counting meditation*. You can also gaze at an object without thinking about it in words. A small object is best, such as a candle, a piece of wood, a stone, or something else you think is appropriate.

To begin the process, find a quiet and relaxing spot, somewhere no one will disturb you. Sit up straight, but relaxed, in a chair, with your forefingers and thumbs touching, palms facing up. (Or, if you prefer, you can choose a moving meditation. For example, you can meditate while you walk, saying, "Right, left, right, left . . .") Body and hand position are important because they act like cues to prepare you to enter the meditation process once you've assumed the position a few times. Just holding your hands as described and directing your breathing gradually toward your abdominal area when you start to feel anxious can often put you into a meditative state, but only if you've put in the requisite practice in a non-anxious state. This can come in handy when you are in a stressful work or social situation and you don't have time to meditate, unless you can graciously excuse yourself and take a bathroom break.

No matter what type of meditation you choose, thoughts will intrude on your meditation process, but with practice, these will decrease. Be compassionate with yourself. This is a technique that you will learn if you persist. As soon as you notice your attention has strayed, gently bring it back to the word or object you are focusing on. Don't spend even an instant on your daydreams or on berating yourself for not staying focused. Never allow meditation to become a race to the finish. Think of meditation as more like a graceful dance.

Learning to meditate is like learning to do anything. It takes time to learn a skill like meditating. Try meditating for just three or four minutes when you start. An easy way to start is to count on the exhale. This would go something like: inhale . . . say the word *one* . . . inhale . . . say the word *two* . . . and so on. Focus on feeling the breath pass through your nose or mouth. If you lose count, try, "In one, in two, in three," and so on. Just enjoy the process and let go of any thoughts that intrude. You might even want to picture them—your thoughts—floating past you in a gentle stream. Later, when you've learned the process, you can meditate for four seconds or four hours.

Another easy meditation is to count your breaths while you perform a task. Choose a simple task like washing dishes, brushing your teeth, scrubbing vegetables, or making a salad or tea. Once you master this meditation, try counting breaths through more difficult tasks like cooking a meal, driving, or enduring a boring meeting.

Use the *walking meditation,* counting a breath each time you take a step, while you're doing errands, cleaning the house, or walking to a potentially stressful meeting. You can also use the walking meditation when you're out for a walk in the country.

When you've mastered these, you may choose to use a *mantra meditation* such as saying the word *om* or *aum* or *amen*, or *blessings,* or *peace.* If you're religious, you can also consult with your minister, priest, rabbi or other religious leader about religious mantras to use.

If you're an artistic person, you might do well with *flame meditation.* Light a candle in a darkened room. Sit a foot away from the candle and stare at it. Blow it out, and with your eyes closed, let the image of the candle come into your mind.

You can increase intimacy and closeness with another person using the *"Ahhh" breath.* Sit with a friend, partner, or patient. Try to match your breathing pattern exactly to your partner's. On exhale, release your breath with an "Ahhh" sigh. This meditation promotes a strong feeling of connection and compassion. It also builds trust and can be used to enhance a relationship.

A *centering meditation* can help you feel more balanced and secure. Stand up straight, with your arms at your sides. Lean forward an inch or two, noticing the tension as your toes dig into the floor. Come back to center. Lean backward an inch until you sense your weight hovering over your heels. Do the same action to the right and then to the left. If you are in a situation where you feel unbalanced, try this centering meditation, but using only very subtle movements forward, back, left, and right.

If you overeat when you're anxious, *conscious eating meditation* may be for you. Take a moment before you begin to eat to clear your mind by counting a few breaths, then focus your attention on picking up your fork, putting food on your fork, transporting the food to your mouth, chewing, noticing the taste, swallowing, and then returning the fork to your plate. If you prefer, concentrate instead on the sensations of the fork in your hand, the sensation of the fork in your mouth, the sensations of the food in your mouth, and so on.

If you are worried or fearful about driving, *conscious driving meditation* may be useful. Instead of worrying, focus your attention on getting into your car, fastening your seat belt, starting the engine, driving down the driveway, the speed of your car, road signs and road conditions. And notice the distance other cars are from you.

You can make almost any activity a meditation if you focus your attention on it—from taking a shower, to shaving, to putting on makeup or getting dressed. Try completing some of these tasks, excluding the shaving and makeup, using your nondominant hand (the left hand if you're right-handed). This will help balance your brain as well as keep you calm.

The benefit of meditation is that it shows you that anxiety is not permanent, that it passes into and out of your body without leaving a trace. When you focus on what is happening right now, the extreme highs and lows of your emotional response to life will disappear and you will live in relative calm.

▪ Panic Diary

If you find yourself panicking, a panic diary may be for you. Each time you have a panic attack, record it. Be sure to include what triggered it, the time of day it occurred, what you were doing at the time, the physical symptoms that accompanied the attack, what you did to cope, what thoughts passed through your head during the attack, and how you would rate the attack in intensity (from one to ten). See the example below of how Toni used her panic diary.

Panic Diary

July 20

Triggering event: My boss yelled at me at 5 P.M., just as I was leaving, claiming I lost a report, which he lost.

Setting: My boss called me into his office.

My reactions: I started to hyperventilate, my heart raced, and my body shook. I thought I was going to faint.

What I did to cope: I felt like screaming, but I counted to ten and waited.

What went through my head: This is never going to end and I'm going to have a heart attack if he doesn't stop talking.

How I'd rate the intensity: I'd rate this a nine out of ten in intensity. It was really bad.

After Toni used this diary form for a while, she began to notice patterns in how she coped, and in what happened. Based on her evaluation, she used progressive relaxation to learn how to quiet her body and not overreact to her boss.

∎ Paradoxical Approach

Although you may want to escape from uncomfortable feelings or fight them, you can achieve even more control by inviting the symptoms. Here are some ways to use paradoxical approaches:

- Invite your symptoms while you're driving, by tensing and relaxing your body.
- When you're at home and on a padded surface, collapse into the soft padding. This approach has been used successfully by many clients who fear collapsing in public.
- To reduce the urge to escape from feared situations, schedule planned exits at crucial times, or stay in the situation a bit longer, asking yourself, "What would happen if I stayed a bit longer?"
- If you have a fear of making a social faux pas, plan ways to commit one, but in a relatively safe way, such as introducing yourself by the wrong name, or going into a clothing store and asking if they sell clothing.
- Return to the scene of a panic attack. This will remove the fear of the place.

∎ Progressive Relaxation

Progressive relaxation is a simple and effective method of systematic deep-muscle relaxation. It has been widely used for many years to counteract the effects of anxiety. It has been shown in a systematic research study to work very well for panic. Progressive relaxation places emphasis on a slow, disciplined development of muscle-tension awareness, providing a powerful weapon against stress symptoms.

Follow the guidelines below and see if they work for you. It may take several tries to obtain relief. You can also purchase relaxation tapes (see the Resources section in the back of this book) or make your own (see below).

According to Dr. Herbert Benson, author of *The Relaxation Response*, a seminal work on anxiety, by going through groups of muscles in turn, tensing them for a few seconds, and very gradually releasing the tension, deeper than normal levels of muscle relaxation can be attained. As well as deepening physical relaxation and heightening our awareness of areas and levels of tension, this technique reliably elicits the "relaxation response" and fosters a more general state of mental and emotional calm. It may take you a few attempts to master the basic procedure, but once you do, your muscles can be relaxed very rapidly. For a greater effect, start with progressive relaxation and combine it with imagery and self-hypnosis (see below).

1. Lie flat on your back, or sit in a comfortable chair. Repeat each of the following steps at least twice. Each session should take about 20–30 minutes.
2. Raise your right leg a few inches off the floor. Arch the foot back and tense the muscles in the leg. Focus on the tension in your leg muscles. Hold (for about 5 seconds) before relaxing (about 20 seconds). Notice the contrast between tension and looseness.
3. Repeat step 2 with the left leg.
4. Repeat with both legs at once.
5. Make a fist with your right hand. Focus on the tension in your right forearm. Hold it for 5 seconds, then relax it. Notice the contrast between tension and looseness.
6. Make a fist with your right hand and bend the arm at the elbow, tightening your biceps. Hold for 5 seconds, then relax. Notice the contrast between tension and looseness.

7. Repeat steps 5 and 6 with the left arm.
8. Repeat with both arms at once.
9. Hunch both shoulders and tense your neck and shoulders. Hold for 5 seconds, then relax. Notice the contrast between tension and relaxation.
10. Raise your eyebrows as far as you can. Hold for 5 seconds. Imagine your forehead muscles becoming smooth and limp as they relax.
11. Squeeze your eyelids shut. Hold for 5 seconds, then relax.
12. Clench your jaw. Bite your teeth down for 5 seconds, then relax.
13. Take a deep breath and hold it for 5 seconds, feeling the tension in your chest and stomach. Exhale and relax completely.
14. Imagine a wave of relaxation slowly spreading throughout your body, starting at your head and gradually penetrating every muscle group all the way down to your toes.
15. Defocus your eyes completely and soften all of the muscles around the eyes. Let the eyes become completely still, passive, and inert.
16. Count softly, out loud, from 1 to 5. Repeat, but twice as softly and slowly. Repeat several times, gradually fading away your voice completely.
17. Do nothing. Notice any sensation in your mouth, tongue, throat, breathing muscles. Let the muscles become completely still, passive, and inert.
18. Remain completely still in this position for about 10 minutes.
19. When you're finished, take a deep breath, stretch your arms, and slowly begin moving.

Making a Relaxation Tape. One of the best ways to learn to relax is to develop your own relaxation tape. Making your own tape allows you to delete segments that don't work for you and to emphasize what is most helpful. You can also add your own music or sound, and develop your own unique approach that includes relaxation comments and coping statements, or images that you find especially peaceful and calming. When you don't have the time or energy to perform your own relaxation procedure, just pop in your specially made tape, lie back, and listen.

Follow these guidelines:

1. **Experiment with your voice.** Speak at normal volume in a flat, almost monotone voice to evoke a hypnotic, relaxing response.
2. **Decide whether you want to add music.** Some composers to consider are Debussy, Bach, Pachelbel, Haydn, and Sibelius. If you like New Age music, consider Steve Halpern, Andreas Vollenweider, and Will Ackerman.
3. **Plan to add some affirmations.** As you relax, you will be in a very suggestible state. Listening to your relaxation tape is the ideal time to hear important affirmations and words that can encourage coping and suggest new and more healthy attitudes. Some helpful affirmations to consider are:

My muscles are beginning to relax, and I can relax them even more.

I am becoming more and more relaxed.

I can stay calm and think about what I need to do. I am in control.

I can relax away my anxiety.

I breathe deeply and calmly when I feel anxious.

Whenever I feel anxious, I fill my body with peaceful light.

Anxiety can't really hurt me; I can stay calm and it will pass.

I can stay calm and go wherever I want.

I can stay calm and breathe slowly.
I can stay calm and focused.
I can relax and feel safe.

Picturing yourself relaxed and calm can make your affirmations more powerful. You may wish to add comments such as, "I picture myself staying calm and going wherever I want."

4. **Writing your relaxation script.** I've included a sample relaxation script below. You can use all or part of it. Pause whenever you see an ellipsis (. . .). Just turn on your recorder and read the words you choose into it. Try it for a time or two. If you don't like it, you can change the script and rerecord until you have the script that works best for you.

Find a quiet spot where no one will disturb you. Loosen your clothing. Take off your shoes. Lie down and close your eyes . . . Focus on your breathing. Let your breath slowly move toward your navel, the center of your body . . . Each time you exhale, let go of whatever it's time to let go of . . . Perhaps as a color . . . Each time you inhale, bring in peaceful, relaxing energy . . . Perhaps as a different color . . . Feel your body becoming more and more relaxed with each breath . . . The next time you inhale, feel your feet filling up with peaceful, relaxing energy . . . Your feet are filling with peaceful, relaxing energy . . . The next time you inhale, fill your lower legs with peaceful, relaxing energy . . . Your lower legs are filling with peaceful, relaxing energy . . . The next time you inhale, fill your knees, front, back, and sides with peaceful, relaxing energy . . . Your knees are filling with peaceful, relaxing energy . . . The next time you inhale, fill your upper legs and thighs with peaceful, relaxing energy . . . Your upper legs and thighs are filling with peaceful, relaxing energy . . . Feel the layers of muscle in your thighs relaxing . . . layer . . . by layer . . . by layer . . . Your legs and thighs are filling with peaceful, relaxing energy . . . The next time you inhale, fill your buttocks with peaceful, relaxing energy . . . Your buttocks are filling with peaceful, relaxing energy . . . The next time you inhale, fill your back with peaceful, relaxing energy . . . Let peaceful, relaxing energy radiate out from your spine to the sides of your back as the layers of muscles in your back relax and fill with peaceful, relaxing energy . . . Your back is filling with peaceful, relaxing energy . . . Now focus on the front of your body, filling up your groin and lower abdomen with peaceful, relaxing energy . . . Your groin and lower abdomen are filling with peaceful, relaxing energy . . . Now focus on filling up your internal organs with peaceful, relaxing energy . . . Picture your internal organs filling up with peaceful, relaxing energy . . . Picture your internal organs relaxing as they spread out and take all the space available to them, filling with peaceful, relaxing energy . . . Picture your chest relaxing, filling up with peaceful, relaxing energy . . . Your shoulders are relaxing . . . The next time you exhale, let whatever you're carrying on your shoulders run right across your shoulders, down your arms, and out your fingertips . . . Just let whatever you're carrying on your shoulders roll right off your shoulders, down your arms, and out your fingertips . . . Now focus on your neck, feel your neck filling up with peaceful, relaxing energy. Your neck, front, back, and sides are filling with peaceful, relaxing energy . . . Let that peaceful, relaxing energy fill your jaw . . . Unlock your jaw and let it fill with peaceful, relaxing energy . . . Your tongue and teeth are relaxing, filling up with peaceful, relaxing energy . . . The next time you inhale, let that peaceful, relaxing energy flow into your cheeks and ears . . . Your cheeks and ears are filling up with peaceful, relaxing energy . . . Let that peaceful, relaxing energy flow through your nose, letting it relax . . . Let that peaceful, relaxing energy flow through your eyes, and the space behind that, and the space behind that . . . Your eyes are relaxing, filling up with peaceful, relaxing energy . . . Let your eyebrows and eyelashes relax, filling up with peaceful, relaxing energy . . . Let your forehead relax, filling up with peaceful, relaxing energy . . . Let your scalp and hair relax, filling up with peaceful relaxing energy . . . Let your brain relax, filling up with peaceful, relaxing energy . . . Take a moment to scan your body. The next time you exhale, send a wave of relaxation to any areas in your body that need to relax more . . . Send that wave of peaceful relaxation to your body now . . . The next time you exhale, you'll find you're a hundred times more relaxed . . . The next time you exhale, send another wave of relaxation to any place in your body that needs more relaxation . . . Your body is feeling so relaxed and peaceful now . . . You realize that each day, and every hour you are becoming more and more relaxed . . . It is getting easier and easier to relax and feel peaceful . . . All you have to do is breathe calmly and you will feel peaceful and relaxed . . . I can relax away my anxiety . . . I now understand that I can breathe deeply and calmly whenever I feel anxious . . . and peace and relaxation will be the result . . . Whenever I feel anxious, I know I can fill my body with peaceful light and I will feel peaceful and relaxed . . . I now know that anxiety can't really hurt me . . . I can stay calm and it will pass . . . All I have to do is breathe and fill my body with peaceful, relaxing energy . . . I now know I can stay calm and go wherever I want to go, staying peaceful and relaxed, breathing easily and calmly, staying peaceful and relaxed . . . I realize I can stay calm and breathe slowly . . . I can stay calm and focused . . . I can relax and feel safe . . .

▌Quieting Response

The quieting response can help you cope with anxiety. It teaches a tension-reduction skill you can use in most situations that you can find solitude, including at home and in the workplace. This kind of relaxation training, as well as other kinds, can reduce insulin dependence, so if you are taking insulin, be sure to talk with your health-care practitioner about working together to reduce your insulin dosage. Here are the steps to take to achieve the quieting response:

1. Sit or lie in a comfortable position in a spot where you won't be disturbed.
2. Breathe easily for a moment.
3. Slowly lift your arms high above your head, take a deep breath, and hold it.
4. Slowly lower your arms to the floor (or to the sides of your chair, or bed) and go completely limp.
5. Hold your hands in a prayer position, pressing them together until your arm muscles begin to tremble, then breathe out and go completely limp.
6. Take a deep breath and hold it while you let your hands touch your face, then breathe out and let yourself go completely limp.
7. Bring your hands into the prayer position again, but hold them 3 inches apart, noticing the warmth between your hands as you breathe, before bringing your hands to rest at your sides.
8. Imagine the sun warm on the top of your head.
9. Imagine your body as a hollow vessel.
10. Feel the warm sunlight that's shining on your head flowing into the vessel, filling it, beginning with your feet and moving up your legs, your abdomen, and your chest.

11. See the warmth reach your shoulders and spill over to fill your arms and hands.
12. Keeping your eyes closed, focus on an imaginary point in front of you. See it as a ball of warm sunlight, filling your mind like a blank screen. Float along for several minutes.
13. When you're ready, play the activities of your day backward on the screen, observing but not reacting to anything you see.

■ Refuting Irrational Ideas

Refuting irrational ideas is another method to reduce anxiety. All of us engage in almost continuous *self-talk* during our waking hours. Self-talk is the internal language we use to describe and interpret the world. When our self-talk is rational, anxiety is reduced. When it's not, anxiety is increased.

At the root of irrational thought is the idea that something is being done to you. Rational thought is based on a more neutral idea that events occur and you experience them.

According to Dr. Albert Ellis, a cognitive-behavioral theorist who developed a system to attack irrational ideas or beliefs and replace them with more realistic interpretations and self-talk, a common form of irrational self-talk is making statements that "awfulize" experience by making catastrophic, nightmarish interpretations of events—for example, interpreting a momentary chest pain as a heart attack, or a grumpy word from a boss as intent to fire, or silence as negative criticism.

The kinds of statements Ellis considers irrational are:

1. People must be unfailingly competent and perfect in all endeavors.
2. The past determines the present.

3. It's easier to avoid difficulties and responsibilities than face them.
4. Unfamiliar or potentially dangerous situations always lead to fear and anxiety.
5. People are helpless and have no control over what they experience or feel.
6. People are fragile and cannot be told the truth.
7. Good relationships are based on sacrifice and giving.
8. Rejection and abandonment result if you don't try to always please others.
9. There is a perfect love and a perfect relationship.
10. A person's worth is dependent on achievement and production.
11. Anger is bad and destructive.
12. It is bad and wrong to go after what you want and need.

Dr. Ellis developed several guidelines for turning irrational thinking into rational thought. Review them whenever you notice irrational beliefs are taking over. You can also write them down and use them as affirmations.

1. The situation does not do anything to me. I say things to myself that produce anxiety and fear.
2. To say things are other than they are is to believe in magic.
3. All humans are fallible and make mistakes.
4. It takes two to argue.
5. The cause of a problem is often lost in antiquity. The best place to focus attention is on the present and what to do about the problem now.
6. People feel the way they think. It's not the events themselves but the interpretation of events that leads to emotions.

Refuting irrational ideas is a skill that requires practice in the following nine steps:

1. Write down the facts of the activating event, including only observable behaviors, not your thoughts or feelings about what happened.
2. Write down self-talk about the event, including all subjective value judgments, assumptions, beliefs, predictions, and worries.
3. Note which statements are irrational by placing a star in front of them.
4. Focus on the emotional response to the event using one or two words, e.g., *anxious*, *fearful*, *angry*, *afraid*, *hopeless*.
5. Select one irrational idea to refute.
6. Write down all evidence that the idea is false.
7. Write down the worst thing that could happen if what is feared happens.
8. Write down what positive effects might occur if what you fear happens or if what you desire doesn't occur.
9. Substitute alternative self-talk.

Tom, a forty-two-year-old lawyer, worked in a law practice. He complained of having to report to one of the partners who made poor decisions and was irresponsible. He agreed to try to refute his irrational ideas so he could sleep at night and not be bothered by repetitive worries. He produced the following information.

1. *Activating event:* My boss humiliates me, and whatever I do is not good enough.
2. *Rational ideas:* I know he's under a lot of pressure because he's new to the job.
3. *Irrational ideas:* I can't stand being humiliated in public. My anxiety takes over and I fear I'll fall apart.

4. *Main feelings:* anxiety, helplessness, anger.

5. *Refuting the irrational ideas:* I'll fall apart.

6. *The worst thing that could happen:* I could tremble or whimper or go speechless.

7. *Good things that could happen:* I can learn how to handle a humiliating boss.

8. *Alternate thoughts:* I'm okay. It's okay to feel anxious and know I can still function. I can learn to handle this situation and feel good about myself for doing so.

9. *Alternative emotions:* I'm anxious, but not out of control. My anxiety is starting to fade and I'm feeling calmer.

■ Self-Hypnosis

Self-hypnosis is a wakeful state of deep relaxation. During hypnosis there is an alteration in the conscious level of your thinking and remembering, and an increase in your ability to focus on a particular situation. Hypnosis is also a heightened state of awareness during which you're more open to suggestion.

You've probably experienced a hypnotic state while daydreaming, or concentrating intently on a task (reading a book, watching a movie or TV program, driving or completing a work project). All hypnosis (including guided hypnotherapy) is really self-hypnosis because you won't accept a suggestion unless your really want to.

During hypnosis you choose to suspend disbelief, just as you do when you become absorbed in watching a movie or TV program. But more than that happens. When you watch a violent chase scene in a movie, your mind and body react as if you were actually participating in the scene. Your muscles tense, your heart rate increases, your stomach knots, you feel excited or afraid. Even your brainwave patterns suggest that you are participating in an activity, although you're just imagining yourself in the activity.

Effectiveness of Self-Hypnosis

Self-hypnosis has been clinically effective with nervous tics, tremors, chronic muscular tension, minor anxiety, and the symptoms associated with anticipatory anxiety (rapid heartbeat; cold sweaty palms; knotted stomach).

Contraindications

If you're disoriented because of organic brain syndrome or psychosis, mentally retarded, or paranoid, hypnosis is not recommended.

Self-Hypnosis Directions

Follow the steps below to practice self-hypnosis:

1. Find a candle, a picture, a crack in the ceiling, a fire in the fireplace, or some other object to use to encourage eye fixation.
2. Preselect a word or phrase to use at the moment your eyes close. The words *relax now*, or the name of a color or a place that is beautiful and has a special meaning for you can also be used.
3. Close your eyes and sit in a comfortable, quiet place where you won't be interrupted. Starting with your toes, tighten and then relax them. Move up your feet to your legs and all the way up your body, first tightening and then relaxing the body part.
4. While watching the object you chose, imagine that your eyes are getting heavier and heavier, are beginning to sting, or are starting to flutter (whichever works best to induce eyelid heaviness.) You can also tell yourself, "My eyelids are getting heavier and heavier." When your

eyelids close, don't forget to say your preselected phrase.

5. When you're ready, return from hypnosis, feeling refreshed and relaxed, or drop off to sleep if it's bedtime, suggesting to yourself that you'll wake in the morning feeling relaxed after a good night's sleep.

Using Suggestions

When forming suggestions for yourself, make sure they are positive, direct, and given only when you feel relaxed; use the word *can* instead of *will* if commands don't work for you; phrase suggestions in the immediate future ("Soon the drowsiness will come"), not the present ("I am drowsy"); form a helpful visual image (imagine yourself looking calm and confident) and emotion or sensation (feel the closeness and belonging you'd like if your anxiety is related to relationships); and avoid saying the word *try* (which implies doubt and the possibility of failure).

Use key suggestions to help you relax. Try each one and see which work for you.

- *drifting down, deeper and deeper*
- *feeling lighter and lighter*
- *drifting and drowsy, so tired* I *can't keep my eyes open*
- *letting myself sink deeper and deeper into my chair (into the floor)*

Write down your suggestions, memorize them, and use a key word to remind you of them when you're anxious. Here are some ideas:

- For obsessive thoughts: *Very soon I will let go of these thoughts.* (Visualize a screen and see the date written there, or see the thoughts being erased.)

- For self-criticism and worry about making mistakes: *I can take a deep breath and let go. I can breathe in positive energy and breathe out whatever it's time to let go of.*
- For low self-esteem: *Everyday I can feel more confident and self-assured. I can be kind to myself. I like myself more and more.*
- For muscle tension: *When I am ready, I can let go and relax my muscles. The sun shines down warm and comforting on my body, helping me relax.*
- For anxiety about an upcoming situation: *I can remember to breathe deeply and say to myself, "Calm and alert." My mind is becoming more and more calm and focused.*
- For performance problems: *I can stay calm and in control. Nothing can upset me. I can imagine myself performing perfectly.*
- For feeling uncomfortable in front of other people: *I can feel relaxed and at ease around other people. I can respond to other people in a relaxed and assertive way. When I put my fingers together, I feel confidence flowing through me.*

A Ten-Minute Self-Hypnosis

Follow the steps below to put yourself into self-hypnosis.

- Touch your thumb to your index finger. Imagine yourself feeling exactly as you do after playing tennis, jogging, walking briskly, or some other exhilarating activity.
- Touch your thumb to your middle finger and take yourself back to a time in your mind, body, and spirit when you had a loving experience.
- Touch your thumb to your ring finger and imagine yourself receiving the nicest compliment you've ever received. Allow yourself to fully accept the words, knowing you are paying that person a compliment in return.

- Touch your thumb to your little finger and imagine the most beautiful spot you have ever seen. Stay there for a while, taking in the sounds, sensations, and view.

■ Systematic Desensitization

Systematic desensitization is a method you can use to reduce your reaction to upcoming situations that you're worried about. This procedure can help you construct a staircase of situations leading up to the upsetting event by breaking it down into its component steps. In this way you can make any situation more manageable. For example, if you are extremely anxious about speaking up in a conference, you might construct the steps between waking up the morning of the conference to the actual moment of speaking. The hierarchy might look something like this:

1. Waking up.
2. Remembering a conference is scheduled.
3. Driving to work and thinking about speaking up in the conference.
4. Arriving at work and seeing the conference schedule.
5. Noticing it is time for the conference.
6. Entering the room where the conference will be held.
7. Sitting down in the conference room.
8. The conference begins.
9. Getting ready to say something during the conference.
10. Speaking in the conference.

Follow the four steps below to use systematic desensitization.

Step 1. Choose an anxiety-provoking situation for which you'd like to use systematic desensitization from the

list below or come up with your own. One way to
choose is to rank the situations from 1 (most distressing) to 14 (least distressing).

___ saying no
___ asking others to tell me what they expect from me
___ praising others
___ telling others what I expect from them
___ taking a compliment
___ admitting a mistake
___ asking for help
___ telling others about their mistakes or limitations
___ standing up for my rights
___ disagreeing with others
___ expressing anger
___ dealing with the anger of others
___ handling a put-down or teasing
___ asking for a legitimate limit to my workload

Step 2. Choose the situation you wish to work on and construct 10 steps (see sample hierarchy above) from least
anxiety-provoking (1) to most anxiety-provoking (10).

1. _____
2. _____
3. _____
4. _____
5. _____
6. _____
7. _____
8. _____
9. _____
10. _____

Step 3. Now think about being in step 1 of the situation you choose. Visualize the situation in your mind. If you experience no anxiety, think about the situation in step 2. If you begin to feel anxious, stop and practice deep breathing and muscle relaxation (see chapter 9). Avoid moving to the next step in the hierarchy until you feel no anxiety when thinking about the step you are focusing on. Continue up the hierarchy until you feel no anxiety when thinking about all the steps you listed.

Step 4. Begin to try this process in real-life situations. Use the same procedure described in step 3.

▌ Thought Stopping

Thought stopping is an approach that is especially useful when nagging, repetitive thoughts make you feel anxious. Cognitive therapist Dr. Aaron Beck uses the term *automatic thoughts* to describe thoughts that are negative and illogical but are still believed, experienced as spontaneous, couched in terms of "should" or "ought," or predict catastrophe or the worst possible result. Such thoughts are persistent and self-perpetuating, based on a unique way of viewing a situation; they repeat habitual themes (for example, danger) that result in tunnel vision and make it impossible to see situations in other ways. Often they are learned in childhood and conditioned by family or friends, or even the media.

There are a number of patterns of limited thinking that create anxiety and that could be reduced or even overcome by thought stopping. I'll discuss seven of them here.

Filtering occurs when you only hear part of a message. For example, your boss tells you the report is good but that next time you ought to make it shorter. In filtering, you only hear the negative comment, blow it up out of proportion, and then think that you're going to be fired for writing a too-long report.

Polarized thinking occurs when you see everything in black and white with no room for shades of gray or even one mistake. If you're a perfectionist and someone criticizes you or your work, you will begin to get down on yourself and your anxiety will soar.

Mind reading is based on the false idea that you can tell what other people are thinking, especially about you. This can raise your anxiety when you interpret a cough or a raised eyebrow as a sign you're disliked or that you did something wrong.

Overgeneralization occurs when you take one incident and assume all others are the same. You reach a conclusion based on only one case. For example, you're overgeneralizing when one person doesn't like your drawing and you assume no one could possibly like it. This can lead to low self-esteem and subsequent anxiety.

Magnifying can occur when you enlarge small things way beyond their true importance, especially anything that implies in any way that you're not perfect. A small mistake becomes a fatal tragedy in your mind and your anxiety increases.

You're *catastrophizing* when you get a stomachache and you're sure it's an ulcer requiring surgery. You read a newspaper report of someone's death or hear about some other problem and start wondering what if that happened to you.

Personalization occurs when you compare yourself with other people and conclude your worth is questionable, or you assume everything others do or say is in reaction to you, or if you constantly test your value and come out on the short end.

See how many limited-thinking patterns you can identify in Tom's story:

Tom came to me because he identified his wife as the source of much of his anxiety. "I keep thinking how smart and cute my wife is and that by comparison I'm a real dope. I know she loves me, but when she gets that look on her face, I know she doesn't like me very much and I worry our marriage is over. Yesterday she told me I did a good job on the toilet handle I put in but that it sticks a little. I feel like she doesn't appreciate one thing I do. I really worked on that handle and now I don't want to do anything around the house anymore.

These kinds of automatic thoughts usually precede anxiety. If you've tried to listen for your automatic thoughts or tried to record them and have been unsuccessful, thought stopping may help you.

The first technique to try when using thought stopping is just to count the negative thoughts you have. Don't do anything to stop them. You can get a knitting stitch-counter or golf stroke-counter and keep track of them. This will help you get some distance from your negative thoughts. Just count the thought and then say, "I release that thought. It is no longer part of me."

Another thought-stopping method is to set a timer for twenty or thirty minutes. When you hear the timer ring, stop what you're doing and pay attention to your thoughts. If you're having negative thoughts about yourself or someone else, count the number and type of negative thoughts. You can write them down in a journal if you prefer, or simply picture releasing the negative thought(s), perhaps as a color.

When using thought stopping, you can also use the command "stop," an image of the letters for the word stop, a loud noise (such as a buzzer or bell), or a negative stimulus, such as wearing a rubber band around the wrist and snapping it when the unwanted thought occurs.

Stella owned her own editing business. She worked out of her home office but occasionally had to go out to meet with clients. It was on those visits that her anxiety skyrocketed. She also reported extreme anxiety when on dates or at social occasions. I taught her several anxiety-reduction techniques, but she reported that thought stopping, especially wearing a rubber band around her wrist and snapping it when an anxiety-provoking thought occurred, worked best for her. She even taught several of her friends the technique. During one of our sessions she reported that they called me "Dr. Rubber Band."

Thought stopping may work because (a) distraction occurs, (b) the interruption behaviors serve as a punishment and what is punished consistently is apt to be inhibited, (c) it is an assertive response and can be followed by reassuring or self-accepting comments, and (d) it interrupts the chain of negative and frightening thoughts leading to negative and frightening feelings, thus reducing anxiety.

For effective mastery, regular practice for three to seven days is needed. Other guidelines include:

- Choose the problematic thought.
- Bring the thought to attention.
- Close your eyes and imagine a situation during which the anxiety-provoking thought is likely to occur.
- Interrupt the nagging thought with an egg timer, alarm clock, snap of the fingers, image, or verbalization of the word *stop*, or by snapping a rubber band you wear around your wrist.
- Replace the nagging thought with a positive, assertive statement, for example—

  For anxiety about being in a group: "I am confident in my ability to remain calm while participating in a group."

  For anxiety about being criticized: "I can listen to negative criticism, determine if it applies to me, and stay calm the whole time."

  For anxiety about turning people down: "I have the right to say no and feel good about it."

For anxiety about making a mistake: "I am human and will
make mistakes, and that's okay."

For anxiety about getting into an argument: "It takes two people
to argue. If I remain calm, there will be no argument."

For anxiety about going after what I want: "I deserve happiness
and reward."

▮ Touch

Touch can be therapeutic. Without touch, babies don't survive for
long. Adults need comforting touch, too. A study published in the
journal *Clinical Nursing Research* found that touch reduced anxiety
in older adults. Touch can calm and soothe. Find a source of safe
touch and ask that person for a hug when you need one.

▮ Uncovering Core Beliefs

Core beliefs are beliefs you've probably held since childhood, or
even longer. They are so much a part of you that you may not even
know you have them. This section will help you uncover core beliefs
that may be increasing your anxiety.

Here are some examples of unhealthy core beliefs:

- Life is dangerous and I have to spend most of my time
  worrying about many dangers.
- I must be perfect at all times and in all ways.
- I'm very vulnerable and cannot deal with too much stress.
- I may pass out or have a heart attack, if my anxiety is high.
- I can't cope with unexpected or anxiety-provoking situa-
  tions.

- Unusual sensations in my body are always a sign that something terribly wrong is happening.
- If I feel anxious, there must be a good reason for it.

One of the things you may notice about all these beliefs is that they are blanket statements. They are absolutes. They leave no room for in-betweens or exceptions. They are so strict, they can increase your anxiety and make change appear hopeless.

Can you alter such strong core beliefs? You can if you're willing to follow the suggestions below to help you get to your core beliefs.

1. Start with an anxiety-related automatic thought—for example: What if I can't control myself?
2. State this as a theory—for example: I may lose control.
3. Be more specific—for example: I may lose control and act like an idiot.
4. Explain why that is a problem for you—for example: If I lose control, people will think I'm an idiot.
5. Tell why if people think you're an idiot, you'd be upset—for example: If people think I'm an idiot, maybe I *am* an idiot.
6. Tell why that would create anxiety for you—for example: Maybe I am defective.
7. Tell what it would mean to you to be defective—for example: I couldn't work anymore, my wife would leave me, and my life would be over.
8. And then what?—for example: And then I'd probably end up in the nut house.
9. How long have you had this belief?—for example: Since I was ten, when my father ended up in the nut house, and I probably inherited his genes.

The core belief could just as well be that you have to carry the burden of unrelenting anxiety throughout life because you were molested as a youngster, that you are destined to be anxious and un-happy, that people can never be trusted, or that you'll freak out if you have to perform a task. The core belief might have been formed in a preverbal state, and may never have been named or discussed. To begin to change core beliefs, start with affirmations (near the beginning of this chapter) that counter your negative thinking. You can also use imagery and thought stopping (also discussed above).

■ Worry List

Start a worry list by writing down all the things you worry about. Beside each one, write down two ways you can handle that worry. Decide which way you prefer to handle each item on your list and set a time frame. Once you get your worries out on the table and start problem-solving about how to deal with them, you'll find it easier than you thought to stop worrying.

■ Summary

This chapter has presented many anxiety-reducing techniques. Choose several approaches from the following list of self-care healing measures and see how they work for you. If your anxiety is still bothersome, return to the list and choose a few more actions. Work along until you find the combination of approaches that helps you the most.

- Accept Your Anxiety
- Act "As If"
- Acupressure or Acupuncture
- Affirmations
- Alexander Technique

- Autogenics
- Breathing Awareness
- Chromotherapy
- Coping Skills
- Focus on the Now
- Imagery
- Inner-Directed Movement
- Journaling (Journal Writing)
- Massage
- Meditation
- Panic Diary
- Paradoxical Approach
- Progressive Relaxation
- Quieting Response
- Refuting Irrational Ideas
- Self-Hypnosis
- Systematic Desensitization
- Thought Stopping
- Touch
- Uncovering Core Beliefs
- Worry List

10

Relationships, Purpose, and Spirituality

The ability to understand and not be upset by other people in your life is crucial to reducing anxiety, as is your relationship to yourself, your life, and a Higher Power (or God). In this chapter, you'll find information about how to feel better about yourself, reduce sources of interpersonal anxiety, and be more assertive, empathic, purposeful, and spiritual.

▮ Self-Esteem and Self-Sabotage

Self-esteem is an ongoing evaluation of yourself and your abilities. Self-esteem reflects your confidence in what you say or do. Feeling sabotaged can result in anxiety. You thought you could trust a colleague, family member, or friend, but you found out you couldn't. It may feel like a knife in the back—or in the heart. You may panic and think you'll never get over such treatment. It's important to realize that everyone has this experience sometimes, and that you must start again and not hide from it.

It may be that no one is sabotaging you but you. Why would you want to sabotage yourself? Low self-esteem is one explanation. When you have low self-esteem, you probably have difficulty standing up to other people, avoid eye contact, turn red easily, and get a "shame attack."

If you have low self-esteem, it is probably because you weren't valued by your caregivers when you were a child. They did not esteem you in an appropriate way. In neglecting to value you, they abused you, even if they didn't mean to. This led to a lack of confidence about yourself and your worth. Low self-esteem can make you feel as if you'll never be able to cope with your anxiety.

Because you may have been abused or neglected in your family of origin, you may abuse or neglect yourself. The key to elevating your esteem is the willingness to take responsibility for your thoughts, feelings, and actions.

Self-esteem fluctuates depending on your life experiences. If you have low self-esteem, take heart. You can learn to build your self-esteem, but it won't happen overnight.

When you make the decision to value yourself, it will be easier for you to value others. As your self-esteem rises, so will your esteem of others. This change will improve your relationships.

On the surface, you may think you want to succeed, but when you have low self-esteem, old messages you learned in your family continue to operate. Perhaps you were told you were stupid, lazy, would never succeed, or were given some other negative message. These messages are like tapes that play in your head. They're faulty because they have nothing to do with you and everything to do with the person who gave you the message. The faulty messages may even seem automatic, as if they can turn themselves on and play and play and there is nothing you can do about it.

There *is* something you can do about these messages, but first you must identify them and realize they are not about you. They belong to someone else. Until you identify these messages, face them, and realize you are worthy and whole, you will continue to sabotage yourself.

Use the exercise below to help identify and eliminate your faulty tapes.

1. Find a quiet, safe spot where you can be alone and undisturbed. You may wish to record the following directions so that you can relax and concentrate on the experience. If you do record them, make sure you read them slowly and in a monotone voice, pausing for several seconds at each ellipsis (. . .).

2. Take a pad and pen with you and sit in a comfortable chair.

3. Kick off your shoes . . . loosen your clothing . . . do whatever you have to do to feel comfortable and safe.

4. Pay attention to your breathing . . . Give yourself a gentle suggestion to let your breath begin to move lower in your body . . . moving toward your center . . . your abdominal area.

5. Picture yourself very young . . . you are back in your family with your parent(s) . . .

6. See yourself in your room . . . hear your parent(s) speaking to . . . or about you . . . What are the words telling you about yourself?

7. Pay attention to the messages that are sarcastic, humiliating, hurtful, or frightening . . .

8. When you have the words well in mind, write down the messages you heard . . . write them all down so you can look at them . . .

9. Examine the list of messages you received from your parent(s) . . .

10. Put a check mark in front of the ones that are behaviors and attitudes you want to keep in your life . . . Release the others . . . seeing them flow away from you . . . no longer able to affect you . . .

11. Repeat this exercise . . . this time . . . write about school experiences that led to your feeling humiliated . . . Take your time . . . Get them all down . . . When you're finished, examine your list and decide which of these attitudes and behaviors you want to keep . . . release the others . . . seeing them flow away from you . . . no longer able to affect you . . .

12. Go back and write about work experiences that led to feeling disempowered . . . Save these answers, too . . . Decide which of these attitudes and behaviors you want to keep . . . release the others . . . seeing them flow away from you . . . no longer able to affect you . . .

▌Hooked on Helping

Helping others can be a positive thing, but when you're hooked on helping, it can intensify your anxiety. You're hooked on helping when you become overinvolved in "taking care of" or "worrying about" others.

If you're hooked on helping, you never learned to separate out your responsibility for your own behavior from taking responsibility for what others do. You probably learned to take care of others early in life. This is common if you came from an abusive family where you were abused by one or both parents, or where one or both parents were addicted to alcohol or drugs. It's also common in a family where one member needs a lot of care and you were designated (by yourself or someone else) the one to take care of that person, even though it is inappropriate for a child to be made responsible for what happens to a sibling or parent.

Guilt may have played a role, too. Guilt set in when you started to believe you really were responsible for someone else's behavior, even though you could only be responsible for your own.

Whatever your situation, if you are overly helpful, boundaries between you and others are not clearly defined. You learned early to get so involved with others and their needs that you may have lost your own identity and stopped taking care of yourself in order to help others.

Rate yourself on the boundary questions below.

	Never	Seldom		Sometimes		Often		Always	
1. I can separate other people's feelings and thoughts from my own.	1	2	3	4	5	6	7	8	9	10
2. I believe I am responsible for my own thoughts, feelings, and actions.	1	2	3	4	5	6	7	8	9	10
3. I believe other people are responsible for what they think, feel, and do.	1	2	3	4	5	6	7	8	9	10
4. I am autonomous and independent.	1	2	3	4	5	6	7	8	9	10
5. I can communicate my rationale for what I value and believe.	1	2	3	4	5	6	7	8	9	10
6. I allow others to have their own values and beliefs.	1	2	3	4	5	6	7	8	9	10
7. I ask others when they need help and respect their answer.	1	2	3	4	5	6	7	8	9	10
8. I ask for help when I need it.	1	2	3	4	5	6	7	8	9	10
9. I can negotiate with others to make sure their needs and mine are satisfied.	1	2	3	4	5	6	7	8	9	10
10. I believe all people are of equal value.	1	2	3	4	5	6	7	8	9	10

The more answers you rated 1 through 7, the lower your self-esteem and boundary skills. The more answers rated 8 through 10, the higher your self-esteem and the better your boundary skills. If you have low self-esteem, you will have difficulty taking good care of yourself and may be increasing your anxiety by taking on responsibilities that aren't really yours.

One activity that will help you build appropriate boundaries is learning to say no. You may have come from a family where it wasn't okay to say no, where you had to hide your disagreement or individual choices. Now that you're an adult, you have the right to say no and it's appropriate to do so. Follow the guidelines below to help establish boundaries.

1. Practice saying "No!" or "I don't want to!" in private, aloud, at least twenty times a day. Do this in a safe environment, such as when you're in your car, in the bathroom, or home alone. Also make comments such as "No, I don't want to go to the meeting," or "No, I don't want any of that food," or "No, I don't want to finish this report." Be sure to include statements concerning whatever else you don't want to do.

2. Be aware of anything you choose to do that you don't want to do. Write about these instances in a journal, being careful not to censor what you write.

3. Note anything you're procrastinating about. If it's work, pick it up, look at it, and tell yourself, "It's okay not to want to do this."

After you've learned to say no, begin work on negotiation skills. Remember that relationships are all about negotiation. I wash your clothes, you take me out to dinner. I clean the house inside, you take the car for service. Without negotiation, you can become anxious, angry, and dissatisfied. Use the following guidelines for effective negotiation:

1. State what the problem, or issue is for you, why it's a problem, and what outcome you would like to achieve. For example, "I get anxious when you stay out late and don't call. I would like you to call me whenever you're going to be home late."

2. Ask your partner what outcome he or she would like to achieve and why.

3. Suggest as many options as you can that would help you both get the results you want.

4. Ask your partner for more options.

5. Reach an agreement, write it out (including who will do what, and when).

6. Negotiate a penalty clause: what each of you will do if you do not honor all aspects of the agreement that you've made. Write this down also.

7. Sign the agreement, and ask your partner to sign, too.

With some important issues, when you can't reach agreement, you may have to set an ultimatum; for example, "If you don't come with me for counseling, I will leave the relationship," or "If you don't call when you're coming home late, I won't wash your clothes this week," or "If you keep taking my jewelry without my permission, I'm putting a lock on the box," or "If you don't stop making sexually inappropriate remarks, I'm filing a harassment suit against you."

Your partner doesn't have to agree to your ultimatum. It's a statement of your own boundaries, and of what you will do if they aren't respected. It's best to take into account the needs, feelings, and resources of both of you when making ultimatums.

▌ Assertiveness

Assertiveness is the ability to stand up for your thoughts, feelings, or desires. It means being able to stand up for reasonable rights (while being respectful of others' rights) for setting goals, for acting on goals by following through consistently, and for taking responsibility for the consequences of your actions. Taking assertive action gives you the potential to interact with others as adults (not as adult and child, or parent and child, situations that are more apt to occur during aggressive or avoidant behavior).

Assertiveness includes an active orientation to life. When you're assertive, you don't wait for situations to improve, you take action to improve them. You do your homework and put forth solutions. You work toward using your full potential, and you do it in a self-directed way. You can tell others what you expect and what others can expect from you, remind them of deadlines, of tasks to be completed, and of work toward long- and short-term goals. Being assertive also means you can tell others about your special skills or achievements, not hide your talents and competencies.

When you're assertive, you make clear, concise statements, stick to the issue or problem at hand, and can initiate and maintain a conversation with whomever you choose. Assertiveness also provides an outlet for your tension. When you hold feelings in or avoid them, your anxiety level can rise. That's why it's important to learn assertiveness skills as a way to reduce your anxiety. Being assertive can reduce anxiety because it helps you express your thoughts and feelings directly. This can bring increased feelings of self-confidence, while reducing anxiety and physical complaints, and improving communications with others. Just remember that the purpose of being assertive is not to get what you want but to express yourself in a calm, reasonable, respectful, and direct manner.

What Are Your Rights?

Part of finding out who you are is affirming your rights as a person. You have the following rights:

- You have the right to work in an environment that is physically, emotionally, and spiritually healthy.
- You have the right to change your mind.
- You have the right to judge your own behavior, thoughts, and feelings, and to take responsibility for their initiation and consequences.
- You have the right to participate in policies that affect your work.
- You have the right to choose not to give reasons or excuses for your behavior.
- You have the right to make excuses and take the consequences.
- You have the right to say, "I don't know."
- You have the right to say no without feeling guilty.
- You have the right to find dignity in self-expression and self-enhancement through your work.
- You have the right to be recognized for your contribution by being provided with an environment that is physically, emotionally, and spiritually healthy.
- You have the right to take social and political action to enhance your work situation and consumer treatment.

Assertiveness vs. Nonassertiveness

What's the difference between being assertive and nonassertive? Nonassertive comments blame the other person and don't take responsibility for moving forward. Here are some examples:

Nonassertive Comments	Assertive Comments
You should have called.	• If you're going to be late, please call so we can reschedule.
You don't appreciate me.	• I'd like a written evaluation of my work.
You didn't hear a word I said.	• Please listen to my opinions even if you don't agree with them.
	• I want to talk with you about our discussion yesterday. For me it isn't finished.
	• I want to talk with you about some things that are bothering me.
I never get a chance to add my two cents' worth.	• I want a say in decisions that affect me.
	• I'm starting to feel resentful and I don't want to feel that way, so please let me choose what we do every other time.
We never discuss anything.	• Let's sit down and talk with no interruptions.

Being Assertive Respects the Other Person

Do you think assertiveness is rude? There is no reason for assertiveness to be disrespectful. You can be polite and still be assertive. When you're assertive, you describe the facts without embellishing or manipulating; for example, "I feel upset about being teased," or "I feel angry when I'm not listened to." Once you express your feelings, you can then ask for an action in a polite way, such as, "Please finish your report as we agreed," or "Please acknowledge my contribution to the effort." To add an extra quotient of respect, restate the other person's viewpoint or feelings while maintaining your position; for example, "I hear your anger, but this is important to me," or "I understand this isn't important to you, but I feel better when we finish on time."

I-Messages vs. You-Messages

Being assertive requires taking a risk by clearly stating what is expected from others and what they can expect from you. Examples of I-messages are: "I would like to . . ." "I suggest we settle this by . . ." "I want to focus on working this out," "This is an issue I can't compromise on," "I feel angry when I'm called lazy."

You-messages are aggressive and have an element of control or manipulation. Examples include: "Why didn't you . . . ?" "You should have . . ." "I think you're crazy." Sometimes you-aggressive messages masquerade as assertive ones; for example, "I think you're wrong!" "I feel you ought to change," "I want you to do as I say." In these messages, the speaker tries to control the listener by judging behavior, or by attempting to force a change in action.

Some we-messages can also be assertive, especially if they imply collaboration, such as, "We can meet and work this out." (Undifferentiated messages—such as "Let's do our exercises together," when only one person is exercising—are neither assertive nor collaborative.)

You-blaming messages are also aggressive. They tend to put others on the defensive and shouldn't be used in conversation. Examples of this type of aggressive statement are: "Why didn't you take care of that?" "Why can't you do it right?" "This is your fault," and "Why are you going around upsetting everyone?"

Some assertive messages can use the word *you* while neither blaming nor coercing the other person. Examples include "Would you like to tell me your point of view?" "I want to thank you," and "I thought I heard you say . . ."

Assertive Responses

It's not unusual to confuse assertiveness with aggressiveness. Let's take a look at some assertive responses.

Situation 1: Someone comes up to you while you are in the middle of an important task and asks you for help with something. An assertive response would be: "I'm just finishing this up. I can help you in ten minutes."

Situation 2: Someone you know starts to holler and berate you. An assertive response is: "I don't like to be shouted at, but I'd like to hear what's upsetting you."

Situation 3: You notice a colleague, family member, or friend doing something unsafe. When you begin to talk to her, she accuses you of picking on her. An assertive response would be: "Let's talk about this and straighten things out between us."

Situation 4: A friend, family member, or colleague agreed he would complete a task, but when you check, the task has not been completed. An assertive response would be: "We agreed you'd be finished with the task by now."

Situation 5: Someone catches you in an error. An assertive response is, "You're right. I did make a mistake."

Situation 6: A friend or family member is always signing you up for courses or activities you have no interest in. An assertive response would be: "I appreciate your concern, but I want to make my own decisions."

Nonverbal Aspects of Assertiveness

If your facial expression or posture is nonassertive, it won't matter what you say. That's why you also need to think about what your body is saying. Speaking loudly enough, and in a firm, fluent voice, maintaining good eye contact, and using facial expressions, gestures, body postures, and positioning that match your words are all important if you want to appear assertive. If you pause too often, laugh nervously, look up or down or away, look angry when you claim you're not, overapologize or overexplain, get sidetracked on irrelevant issues, talk too much, don't allow others to speak, use sarcasm, whine, plead, try to make the other person feel guilty, roll your eyes, qualify your statements, or blame the other person, you will not appear assertive.

Strive for a relaxed body posture. It conveys self-confidence, interest, openness, and nondefensiveness. If this is difficult for you, use one or more of the techniques presented in chapter 9.

Facing the person you're speaking to is part of an assertive presentation, as is standing or sitting an appropriate distance away. Being too close or too far away will interfere with being assertive.

Techniques for Enhancing Assertiveness. You can practice by looking in your mirror to give you feedback about whether your words fit with the gestures and your posture. Mirror practice can also be helpful in rehearsing assertive statements prior to trying them in real-life situations. This kind of rehearsal can build confidence so you can be assertive in the real-life situation.

Audio and video recorders also provide excellent practice in assertiveness. Audio recordings provide clues about whether you pause frequently enough, whether your tone of voice is assertive, whether you speak too quickly, and whether you stick with an issue and sound assertive. Some statements to record and evaluate for assertiveness are:

- I see your point but I disagree.
- I made an error.
- I have made my mind up about this.
- I feel angry about this.
- I cannot talk to you now. Let's talk at one o'clock.
- Let's sit down and work this out together.
- This item is not negotiable.
- I'm upset about our relationship and I'd like to talk with you about it.

- I appreciate your help.
- You agreed your report would be on my desk yesterday. What happened?

Video feedback adds additional information about eye contact, changes in body posture and positioning, facial expressions, and confidence of presentation. Probably the best use of video is for rehearsing upcoming situations you think will evoke anxiety. Write a script for a conversation between you and another person. Record it with a friend or colleague and then evaluate whether you're satisfied with your performance or not.

Another way to use video is for *role-playing*. In this approach you tell another person about an upcoming or past situation. (It is best to use a two-person situation; avoid those with a long history of emotional overlay; and strive for choices that are likely to end in a successful role-play, not in frustration.) You will have to coach your partner about the situation, what role each of you will take, how the other person should act to approximate the real-life situation, and how the interchange will begin and end. A three-to-five-minute script is sufficient when extraneous discussions are omitted and you adhere to the main topic. Some directions to give your partner include: "Be sure to try to make me feel guilty about saying no," or "Every time I try to stick to the issue, you change the subject," or "Use a really angry tone of voice, but insist you're not angry."

Using a script and trying it out will help you identify areas that require further practice or more information. For example, if you're asking for a raise, it's necessary to "do your homework," which means spending time thinking about your response and coming up with alternate solutions for the problem that provide adequate information for the other person to support your point of view. You'll have to show your boss exactly what you've done that justifies being rewarded with a raise.

Fears That Prevent Assertiveness

It's important to be aware of which fears may be preventing you from being assertive. Check the fears that inhibit your assertiveness.

___ 1. Fear of rejection

___ 2. Fear of hurting the other person's feelings

___ 3. Fear of being too aggressive

___ 4. Fear of showing my feelings

___ 5. Fear of being unfeminine (or unmasculine)

___ 6. Fear of losing control

___ 7. Fear of learning "the truth" about myself

___ 8. Fear of being retaliated against

___ 9. Fear of being punished by an authority figure

___ 10. Fear of failing and looking silly

___ 11. Fear of _____

Overcoming Your Fears of Being Assertive

To overcome your fears of being assertive you must confront the myths behind them. Let's examine each fear.

- **Fear of rejection.** Although it is possible some people may not like what you have to say, there is no guarantee they'll like you even if you don't speak up. It's impossible to have everyone like you, so you might as well speak up and say what's on your mind.

- **Fear of hurting the other person's feelings.** If you speak assertively, you will be respectful of other's feelings. Although it is possible that some people may not like what you have to say, or even listen totally to what you say, not speaking up means not being truly who you are.

- **Fear of being too aggressive.** If you follow the suggestions in this book and speak in a respectful way, you will not be aggressive.

- **Fear of showing my feelings.** You can choose whether to show your feelings or not. If you prefer, you can focus on the behavior or goal you have in mind and not mention your feelings. If you practice using the suggestions in this chapter, you will learn how to express your feelings without becoming overemotional.

- **Fear of being unfeminine (or unmasculine).** Assertiveness is neither feminine nor masculine. Both men and women can be assertive.

- **Fear of losing control.** It is more common to lose control when you aren't assertive. Holding feelings in and avoiding upsetting situations can lead to blowing up and being aggressive. If you are assertive when a situation happens, you are less likely to lose control.

- **Fear of learning "the truth" about myself.** Being assertive can help you be more yourself, and in a way that is a kind of truth. If you're worried that by being direct you will learn upsetting and potentially damaging information about yourself, that is not likely to happen, although it *can* happen when you hold your feelings in and then blow up at someone else.

- **Fear of being retaliated against.** It is possible not everyone will like what you have to say when you're being assertive, but since you'll be respectful, it is far less likely that others will retaliate than when you're being aggressive.

- **Fear of being punished by an authority figure.** It's always wise to pick your battles. You will need to weigh whether it's worth the possible consequences of being assertive or whether you should find another outlet for your thoughts and feelings.

- **Fear of failing and looking silly.** Failing doesn't have anything to do with being assertive. Your purpose is to express your thoughts and/or feelings. If you can do that in a respectful way, you'll never look silly.

Challenging Counterproductive Beliefs

Once you've identified your core anxieties and fears, you're one step closer to being assertive. It's admirable to strive to handle situations well, but it's counterproductive to expect to change old patterns overnight when you've spent years developing them. Beliefs held by others can end up defeating your attempts to be assertive unless you prepare for them. Many people confuse assertiveness with aggressiveness and may question your interest in becoming more assertive. It's wise to prepare for this type of comment and know some possible ways to respond. Read the counterproductive-belief questions below.

Question: *Why do you want to be assertive? Isn't that just a way of manipulating other people to get what you want?*

Answer: No. Being assertive means standing up for your rights, knowing full well that other people have rights, too. Being assertive is less manipulative than verbal stabs in the back, avoiding important issues, or blowing up with anger.

Question: *If someone gets angry when I'm assertive, isn't that anger my fault?*

Answer: No. You cannot be responsible for someone else's behavior, but you might be able to teach that person how to accept reasonable limits without becoming unduly angry.

Question: *Shouldn't I be able to meet other people's demands and needs as well as my own?*

Answer: Assertiveness is a skill that requires planning, practice, and hard work to master. It's unrealistic to handle situations in a new way spontaneously; that can lead only to frustration and downplaying your potential. You cannot be responsible for anyone else's reactions and feelings, only your own. Being assertive means being able to admit to both strengths and weaknesses. It means being able to say "I don't know" when you don't.

Question: *Shouldn't I be able to be assertive without ever threatening or frustrating other people?*

Answer: It's doubtful the other person is so fragile that your words could produce irreparable damage. Despite how respectful you are, some people may view your behavior as a threat. Just remember you have a fifty-fifty chance that others will respond positively to your assertive action. Chances are quite good that no matter what others do, you will like yourself better if you are assertive. Even if other people get annoyed at you for being assertive, you can handle it. If the other person becomes unreasonably angry, it's doubtful the situation will escalate unless you respond with aggressive words or behavior. Just remember you're responsible only for your own behavior, not the other person's. Also remember that remaining silent and hoping that someone else will handle the situation is avoiding your responsibility.

Question: *Shouldn't I be able to handle situations better than I do?*

Answer: Putting yourself down for not handling situations as well as you would like is a waste of your time and energy. Instead, if you think of a good response you wish you'd said, write it down to use next time. As long as you and the other person are alive, you can work at resolving situations. Once you have in mind the assertive words you want to use, approach the other person and say something like, "I've been thinking about our argument last week and I'd like to talk with you and resolve it," or "Remember that disagreement we had yesterday? I'd like to talk to you about it."

Question: *Won't people think I'm cold and uncaring if I assert myself?*

Answer: It's probably just the opposite, but some people may still accuse you of being cold and uncaring as a way to manipulate you so you'll comply with what they want. Remember you have a right to have your own needs and goals met. Treating other adults as capable people, which is part of being assertive, will enrich a relationship.

Question: *Can I become too assertive so that I overwhelm others?*

Answer: You can't be too assertive. One aspect of assertiveness is that it's appropriate to the situation.

Assertiveness at Work

Being assertive means you have realistic work goals. *Unrealistic* goals include the need to:

- be needed
- be liked
- master impossible tasks or impossible situations
- be the "good child" by winning approval
- have others feel sorry for you

Realistic work goals include:

- making money
- earning a living
- pursuing glory, status, or prestige

- being rewarded for interest or skill
- doing meaningful work
- personal growth and change

Constructive work habits are another part of assertiveness. This means being able to structure a satisfying day, set limits on others' interruptions and requests, concentrate on one task at a time, complete unpleasant tasks without procrastinating, and structure work to reward yourself.

Giving and taking criticism, evaluation, and help is another part of assertiveness. This includes feeling comfortable taking compliments, praising others, owning up to your mistakes or errors, pointing out others' limitations or need for learning, asking for assistance when you need it, and staying calm while being observed or evaluated.

Setting Assertiveness Goals

If you decide to change to more assertive behavior, the first step is to prioritize your assertiveness needs. Take a look at the behaviors below and see which of them are a high priority for you.

Verbal Presentation of Self

____ I make clear, concise statements.

____ I stick to the issue/problem at hand.

____ I initiate and maintain a conversation.

____ I express my thoughts and feelings openly.

____ I use "I" or collaborative "we" statements.

Nonverbal Presentation of Self

____ I speak in a loud, firm, fluent voice.

____ I maintain eye contact.

____ My facial expression is appropriate to my words.

____ My body posture conveys interest and openness.

____ I position myself to sit or stand an appropriate distance from whomever I'm talking with.

Active Orientation

____ I suggest policies, procedures, and solutions.

____ I work to my full potential in a self-directed way.

____ I tell others exactly what they can expect from me.

____ I ask others exactly what they expect of me.

____ I plan short-term and long-term goals.

____ I work to achieve my goals.

____ I tell others of my special skills and achievements.

____ I remind others of deadlines or time frames without nagging or trying to make them feel guilty.

Constructive Work Habits

____ I structure my day so that I am reasonably satisfied with its outcome.

____ I limit other people's interruptions.

____ I concentrate on one task at a time.

____ I find a way to complete unpleasant tasks.

____ I say no to illegitimate requests.

____ I structure my work to reward myself.

Giving and Taking Criticism and Help

____ I can take compliments and feel comfortable.

____ I can praise others for their achievements.

____ I own up to my mistakes and limitations.

____ I point out others' limitations or need for learning in a neutral way.

____ I ask for assistance when I need it.

____ I remain calm when being observed or evaluated.

Control of Anxiety or Fear

I can feel comfortable when . . .

_____ standing up for my rights.

_____ disagreeing.

_____ expressing anger.

_____ dealing with others' anger.

_____ handling a putdown or teasing.

_____ asking for a legitimate limit to my workload.

_____ taking a reasonable risk.

Learning to Say No

One of the most difficult tasks you may face is saying no, especially if you were brought up to please other people and not rock the boat. To be assertive, it's imperative to learn to say no to demands that conflict with your own needs and desires. Saying no effectively also means saying no without feeling guilty. You really have to learn to believe that you have a right to say no and mean it.

In many cases, just saying "No, thank you" or "No, I'm not interested" may be enough. Some people may persist, and that's when it's important for you to repeat your refusal without apologizing. To emphasize that you really mean what you're saying . . .

- look the other person in the eye.
- raise the level of firmness in your voice slightly.
- repeat your refusal—for example; "I said no, thank you."

If you feel compelled to give an explanation, acknowledge the other person's request by repeating it, explain your reason for declining, and repeat your no statement. When it's appropriate, you may wish to suggest an alternative proposal that meets both your needs.

It may help you to say no if you think about what precedes saying no (acknowledgment and explanation), and what can follow saying no (alternative option). Here are some examples to help you say no.

Example 1

"I understand that you want me to get my report in early [acknowledgment], but you gave me two other assignments that you told me must be completed first [explanation], so I have to tell you that the report won't be done early unless I get some help with the other assignments [saying no]. Would you be open to finding someone to help me with those two assignments so that I could get the report in early? [alternative option]."

Example 2

"I hear you need some help with the dishes [acknowledgment]. I'd like to help you but I have schoolwork to do [explanation], so I'm not going to be able to help [saying no]. Maybe Jim can help you [alternative option]."

Keep in mind that you never have to answer a question right away unless it's a life-threatening situation. You can always take your time answering. "Give me a day to think this over," or "I can't answer you right now. I'll get back to you this afternoon," or "I need more information before I can act," or "There may be something in what you say; let me think about this for a few minutes." When the conversation reaches an impasse, but the discussion is an important one, you can delay talking to a later time. This kind of action is only assertive if you set a specific time in the near future to continue the discussion.

Excuses and apologies are often carryovers from childhood when your parents or teachers demanded them. In a few situations, an apology may be relevant, but even then, never overapologize. Just restate the other person's request and explain why you can't meet it. If you imply that you're not sure, that gives the other person ammunition to try to make you feel guilty about saying no. Avoid promising to do something else for the person you say no to. There is no need to feel guilty. You have the right to say no.

Practice using assertive nonverbal communication by looking in a mirror and saying what you have to say. Check to make sure you have good eye contact, keep a confident expression on your face, and use a firm and calm tone of voice.

Challenging Your "Shoulds"

If you want to become assertive, one of the major hurdles to overcome is your "shoulds." If you're a woman, part of who you are is based on socialization into being a female. Messages that many women (and some men) commonly receive in our society are that you "should" think of others first, never brag or tell positive things about yourself, always listen and be understanding, never complain, be attuned to what the other person is thinking and feeling, and be willing to give to others. Another message you may have learned in your family is that you are bad. This can happen when parents don't differentiate between bad behavior and bad child. If as a child you got this kind of message, as an adult you probably still believe there's something wrong with you, not with what you may do. You may have been especially confused if your parents got mad sometimes when you did a certain behavior but didn't at other times. This could have led you to think it's not what you do, it's you. These messages can make you susceptible to guilt induction from authority figures as a child and as an adult.

Family members can try to make you feel guilty by giving you the message "You should do what we ask of you, whenever we ask." This message is rarely given so directly, and is usually couched in other words and behaviors, even sometimes with the insistence that you need not help, while showing you in other ways that you should. For example, "That's okay, I'll be fine, don't worry about me," when you know that person won't be fine, but also that it's not reasonable of him to depend on you to make things fine.

Other "shoulds" may come from your work environment. Your boss my tell you, "You should work overtime; you're needed." Peers may tell you, "You should help me; I can't do this without you."

Whenever anyone tells you that you "should" do something, challenge it by explaining why the suggested behavior is counterproductive to your sense of power. Based on your challenges, decide which of your "shoulds" you will comply with, and then state them in a more assertive way. Study the examples that follow.

Shoulds	Choices
You should stay with me and help me.	I choose to help you.
You should work overtime.	I choose to work overtime.
You should do what your mother says.	I choose to do what my mother says.
You should do this work.	I choose to do this work.

Choose a Situation

It is more difficult to establish new behavior in a complex situation (more than two people involved), in which you are taken by surprise (have to think on your feet). It is also difficult to change behavior in an ongoing relationship that tests you to the limit, probably because you have a history with that person and each time you see her you are reminded of past encounters.

For all these reasons, choose a simple, two-person situation in the beginning. You want to build on success, so make sure the situation doesn't have a long history of negative outcomes, and that it will have no effect on important people or objects in your life. For example, don't pick a situation in which you must confront your boss or another important authority figure. Work up to that with simpler, circumscribed situations such as saying no to a stranger or to the clerk behind the counter of a deli or coffee shop you frequent.

Using Behavioral Contracts

Behavioral contracts can help you be more assertive. They help you structure your behavior in a specific and assertive way. Behavioral contracts are especially useful in family situations, but they can be useful in other situations, too.

Successful contracts include straightforward phrases like "I want," and direct consequences, such as "I will take responsibility for . . ." In a family where curfew is a problem, alternative ways to meet curfew could include calling half an hour early to negotiate a new curfew, coming home at a prearranged hour, averaging curfew times, or coming home one hour early in exchange for the use of the car.

Successful contract negotiation requires that you clearly state your goal; for example, "My husband kisses me goodbye when leaving for work." Keep in mind that it is more constructive to focus on contracts that create new behaviors instead of those that emphasize ending old ones. Just as it's easier to smile more often than it is to stop frowning, it's easier to have one meal a week together with the family than to stop eating out alone.

When writing behavioral contracts, also include a specific reward to follow the desired behavior. Here are some examples of such contingencies:

- When your homework is finished, you can watch TV for one hour.
- In exchange for eating one meal a week with the family, Scott does the dishes for Emily that evening.
- When Sarah obtains a card signed by her teacher indicating that her school assignments have been completed, she can do whatever she wishes after school that day. Her fa-

ther will monitor the contract and her mother promises not to nag him; in return, Sarah's father will be allowed to go out one night a week with his friends.

- When Ben finishes forty-five minutes of exercise, he can watch TV for an hour.
- When Tim completes the agreed-upon report, he can go for a half-hour break or leave work half an hour early that day.

Practicing Assertiveness

The best way to become more assertive is to practice assertive responses in a relatively safe and calm environment. Follow these guidelines for the practice that follows.

1. Identify three situations you wish to practice.
2. Examine any counterproductive beliefs or attitudes you have about this area of assertiveness.
3. Write down the specific types of practice you think will help you achieve your assertive goal, including video-taped replay, role-playing with a trusted other, audiotape practice, or practicing in front of a mirror.
4. Write down a specific way you will evaluate your progress. (Will you ask for feedback from someone else? Review the video and critique your performance? Use some other method?)
5. Identify how you will reward your accomplishment of this goal.
6. Write a behavioral contract for this assertiveness goal.

Handling Difficult Situations

Even if you are assertive, some people won't be assertive in return. Assertiveness only allows you to express yourself. It does not guarantee how others will respond to you. They have the right to choose how to react to you, and sooner or later you'll run into people who put off your request by changing the subject, joking or making fun of what you say, questioning or criticizing your comments, getting emotional or angry, trying to make you feel guilty, or asking why you want what you want.

Luckily there are ways to handle these difficult situations. You'll find some of them below.

Acknowledging Whenever you receive criticism, an assertive response includes acknowledging the critic's comment. Some examples are: (1) "You're right, I am half an hour late for work." (2) "You're right, I did misspell a lot of words." and (3) "Yes, I am late in handing in this report."

Clouding Clouding is a useful technique when you receive criticism you don't agree with. Clouding allows you to hold your ground while continuing to communicate with the other person. This approach requires careful listening to what is being said and finding one thing you can honestly agree with, either *in part, in probability*, or *in principle*. The idea is to agree with the part of the person's statement that makes some sense but don't agree to change.

Other Person: "You're late again. Where are you when I need you?"
You: "That's right. I *am* ten minutes late."

Agreeing in Part This action allows you to agree in part, but not completely.

Other Person: "You always have an excuse for not helping me. What's the matter with you?"
You: "I do have a lot of responsibilities."
Other Person: "You don't seem to be here much anymore."
You: "You're right, I guess it seems that way."

Agreeing in Probability By agreeing in probability, you are able to maintain your right to your own opinion.

Other Person: "Putting on a little weight, aren't you?"
       You: "I may have gained a few pounds."
Other Person: "Time for you to go on a diet."
       You: "You may be right."

Agreeing in Principle Agreeing in principle allows you even more power in the situation.

Other Person: "If you don't study more than you do, you're going to fail."
       You: "You're right, if I don't study, I will fail."

Assertive Probing This response gives you time to determine whether criticism is constructive or manipulative, and clarifies unclear comments. The first step in assertive probing is to listen carefully and isolate the part of the criticism that seems most bothersome to the critic. The next step is to ask the critic, "What is it that bothers you about _____?"

Other Person: "You're not doing a very good job here. Your work is not up to par."
       You: "What is it about my work that bothers you?"
Other Person: "Everyone else is working overtime, but you waltz out of here at five o'clock two out of three nights."
       You: "What is it about my leaving on time when other people work overtime?"
Other Person: "I don't like working overtime either, but the work has to be done. It's not right that you just work by the clock."
       You: "What is it that bothers you when I work by the clock?"
Other Person: "When you leave, someone else has to finish your work. I want you to make sure your work is completed before you leave."
       You: "I see. Thanks for explaining the situation to me."

Broken Record This approach is useful when others do not seem to hear or accept what you say, or when an explanation would provide the other person with an opportunity to continue a pointless discussion. It is especially useful for saying no to others' requests when the other person won't accept your no. In such cases, follow the steps below.

Step 1: Clarify exactly what the limits of behavior are.

Step 2: Formulate a short, specific statement about what is preferred; avoid giving excuses or explanations since they give the other person ammunition to undermine your original statement.

Step 3: Use consistent body language that supports what you say, including maintaining eye contact, standing or sitting erect, and keeping your hands and arms quietly at the side of your body.

Step 4: Repeat the chosen statement calmly and firmly as many times as necessary until the other person realizes there is no negotiation possible. The first few times a statement is said, the other person may give an excuse or attempt to derive a different answer.

Step 5 (optional): Briefly acknowledge the other's ideas, feelings, or wishes before returning to the broken-record statement; for example, "I hear you saying you're upset, but I don't want to work any more overtime."

Other Person: "I just got an opportunity to fly to Aspen to ski. Won't you help me out and switch vacation schedules with me?"

You: "How great for you. *No, I don't want to switch schedules.*"

Other Person: "You mean you're not going to help me? What kind of a friend are you?"

You: "I understand that you're disappointed, but *I don't want to switch schedules.*"

Other Person: "I have to go to Aspen and you're the only one who can help me."

You: *"No, I don't want to switch schedules."*

Other Person: "Boy, you really are hard-hearted. What happened to you lately? You used to be so nice, now suddenly you're Wanda the Witch."

You: *"No, I don't want to switch schedules."*

Other Person: "Boy, you're not going to give on this, are you?"

You: "No."

Content-to-Process Shift When the focus or point of the conversation drifts away from the original topic, the content-to-process shift can be used to shift from the subject being discussed (the content) to what is occurring between the two speakers (the process); for example, "We're off the point now, let's get back to what we agreed to discuss."

Content-to-process shift can involve self-disclosure of current thoughts or feelings; for example, "I'm feeling uncomfortable discussing this now, and I notice we're both tense." This approach is especially useful when voices are raised and anger is present; for example, "We seem to be getting into a battle about this." The trick is to comment neutrally about what you observe so that an attack will not be experienced by the other person.

Joining and Circling the Attacker This approach is derived from the martial art of Aiki, in which the attacked person accepts the attack and turns with it, letting the attacker pass in the direction he or she has chosen. You flow with them, harmonize, become the water, not the rock. This works well with people who yell at you. If you yell back, you maintain the anger.

Joining with the Attacker In this approach you offer to help the other person, refuse to take the attack personally, and objectify the conflict between you. By agreeing with the attacker, you provide surprise and temporarily throw him or her off balance.

Other Person: "What have you done? This is the worst job I've ever seen."

You: "I don't blame you."

Other Person: "What do you mean, you don't blame me?"

You: "It's not up to me to blame anybody for feeling the way they do. You're not pleased, and I can't quibble with that."

Other Person: "But you think your work is up to par?"

You: "It can't be if you're not happy with it. My job is to work with you. Let's see if we can't work on this thing and make it mutually acceptable. What are some of your complaints?"

▐ Empathy

Empathy is the ability to accurately perceive the feelings and meanings of other people. If you don't know what your family, friends, or colleagues mean, that can create anxiety. You'll find some examples of different levels of empathy below. They will help you see where you are with your empathy skills and decide where you want to go.

Empathy provides an emotional mirror for the reflection of other people's feelings. Empathic people learn to use the words and language of those they care about and reflect feelings and ideas back without assuming they know what the other person means (even when it hasn't been stated), or judging what the other person says. Advice isn't given unless it's asked for, and then only if there has been an attempt to solve the problem together. No behavior is labeled ("That's crazy," or "That's irrational"); instead, the tone of voice or mood conveyed by the other person is mirrored. Reflection of what is heard is presented in a tentative manner, such as, "It sounds as if you're really anxious," unless there is no doubt about the matter.

Empathy requires the ability to listen actively and to reflect the essence of the other person's words. Although listening seems simple and passive, it is difficult to avoid trying to solve other people's problems for them, telling them what you would do under similar circumstances, or pooh-poohing the problem by discounting its importance ("What are you worrying about? A lot of people have it worse").

When you listen actively, you make a conscious attempt to listen without any preconceived notions; you try not only to understand the words but also the emotions and body movements of the other person. Active listening is necessary to produce reflective communication that combines the words and emotional content just conveyed by the other person. Reflective communication provides a sounding board that helps other people to clarify their thoughts and feelings and to work out their own solutions.

Here are some examples of *low*, *beginning*, and *high empathy*.

Low Empathy. The other person's feelings are ignored and their full meaning isn't grasped.

Example 1:

You: You should exercise more.

Other Person: Why? I'm as healthy as you are.

You: You'll be sorry when you get older.

Other Person: I'm not going to wear myself out.

You: Did you see who won the game? [*changes subject*]

Example 2:

You: Do you have any information on what's healthy to eat?

Other Person: You want to lose weight? [*makes an assumption*]

You: Yes, but after I eat sometimes I feel tired and crawly. I don't—

Other Person: That's probably nothing. [*interrupting*] You worry too much.

Beginning Empathy. You or the other person conveys an accurate awareness of the obvious feelings and their meaning.

You: I've been worried all day.

Other Person: What's your reaction to this? [*get more information*]

You: Maybe I should go to the doctor and get some pills.

Other Person: You think pills might help. [*reflects your opinion*]

You: Maybe. They didn't help before, but I don't know what else to do. It's really making me nervous.

Other Person: You're really nervous. [*reflects back your statement*]

You: Yeah, I just hope I can find a way not to get so anxious.

High Empathy. You're able to communicate accurately and confidently about the current conspicuous feelings of someone else.

Other Person: I hate it when you complain all the time.

You: You don't like it when I complain. [*reflects feeling tone of the other person with your tone of voice*]

Other Person: Yes. You remind me of my mother. She's always complaining, just like you.

Ways to Develop Empathy

There are three approaches you can use to develop more empathy in yourself or others. The first is to practice paraphrasing what the other person says and to ask that person to paraphrase what you say. You can tape-record what is said and compare it for accuracy. Once you identify a lack of active listening, you are ready to work on enhancing your empathy skills.

Another way to develop empathy is to read more information on empathy and its use and discuss how to identify examples of empathy (or its lack) in future conversations. You can also agree to signal each other (hold up a card, a hand, or some other agreed-upon object) when the other person isn't being empathic.

∎ Relationships and Anxiety

Could your relationships be adding to your anxiety? Find out by answering the questions below. The more *yes* answers you have, the more your relationships may be adding to your anxiety.

___ **1.** My boss is not supportive of me.

___ **2.** My colleagues tease or scold me.

___ **3.** My boss teases me or disrespects my efforts.

___ **4.** I am uncomfortable with at least one past or current relationship.

___ **5.** I have at least one person I must deal with at work who is difficult.

___ **6.** At least one person in my life does not hear me when I try to speak about what bothers me.

No matter how hard you work to reduce your anxiety, it's going to be difficult to achieve if the important people in your life sabotage you. Even if that happens, you can still help reduce interpersonal anxiety. Let's take a look at some statements you could use to gain support from others.

- "I'm working to stay calmer and I could really use your help. Would you be willing to help me by _____ [what you need to stay calm; for example not bugging me so much, letting me make my own decisions, and so forth], and in return, I'll _____ [what you'll do in exchange; for example, wash dishes, go shopping, polish shoes, or whatever].

Call a Meeting

Another way to get others in your life to be more supportive of your efforts to reduce anxiety is to call a meeting and ask each person for support. Scheduling a meeting is a good way to work out difficulties with others. Here are some guidelines for calling a meeting.

1. Settle on a day and time that works for the majority.
2. Convince them, and yourself, of how important this is to you. (Give yourself permission to be the center of attention. You deserve it!)
3. Be persistent when individuals grumble or make excuses for not coming to your meeting.
4. Reassure everyone that *they* can get something out of this meeting, too.
5. Ask each person to write down one thing they'd like to change about their relationship with you and bring it to the meeting. Promise that their concerns will be brought up at the meeting, and that you'll support their right to find a solution if they will help you solve your issue.
6. When the meeting takes place, collect everyone's wishes and place them, along with yours, in a pot or hat. Draw out one wish at a time and spend 10–15 minutes discussing each person's wish and how to achieve it.
7. Tell the group that everyone gets to speak, but one at a time, and no arguing. If you like, ask one of the more assertive individuals to verbally stop people from talking over each other or arguing.
8. Keep drawing cards out of the hat or pot until everyone's problem has been discussed and each person, including you, has at least one possible solution for achieving their wish.

Increase Positive Behaviors

Many couples, friends, and colleagues use statements such as, "Why don't you stop . . . ?" Communication experts suggest that instead of making that kind of statement, each of you compile a list of three specific behaviors you would like to increase in the other person. Compare the following statements:

1. "Why don't you stop talking on the phone so much and get your work done?"
2. "I'd like you to increase the time you spend working with me on this project."

The first statement is critical, while the second has a positive ring to it.

Compile your own list of three behaviors you want the other person to increase. Make sure you use specific statements; for example, "I would like to increase the time we spend working on this project from fifteen minutes to thirty minutes a day."

After you've both compiled your lists, ask if your items are acceptable to the other person. If not, modify them. When you both agree your requests are reasonable, shift your attention to putting each item into action. Because you both agree and because all of the items are stated in positive terms, you're both apt to have increased levels of satisfaction with each other.

Find a Like-Minded Group

You can't change your family, but if none of them is supportive of you, find your own group of like-minded people. Connect with them, spend time with them, and ask them for support for you and your ideas. Once you have this new support group, you won't expect so much from family members anymore because you will have another source of support. This will reduce your tension when you're with your family.

Nurture Your Inner You

Do you think of everyone but yourself? When was the last time you treated yourself to something you like? Just like everyone else, you need nurturing. Once we get to be adults, and sometimes even before that, nurturing from others may stop. That's why you have to develop your own ways of nurturing yourself.

Ask yourself the following questions as a beginning to nurturing yourself:

1. What makes me feel good about myself?
2. How can I make that situation come about?
3. If I set a date to start making that feel-good situation come about, when would be the soonest I'd take some action to make it happen?
4. Who do I trust enough to tell about my feel-good situation?
5. How can I get that person to help provide the feel-good situation?
6. What can I provide for that person in exchange for helping me with my feel-good situation?
7. If I don't need another person to provide my feel-good situation, what is my target date for making it happen?

■ Spirituality

Spirituality has to do with your relationship with a higher consciousness or power. When you are spiritual, you give and receive unconditional love, and do unto others as you would like done unto you. This kind of love is love without judgment and absolute caring for the welfare of another. Think Golden Rule.

According to Leland R. Kaiser, PhD, it is hoarding resources that creates scarcity in the community. He reminds us that we are all traveling through this life together and we must take care of each other, not act like predators. Think about how you can collaborate with another person to see how you can both get what you need and want.

Spirituality is the unifying force, the essence that shapes and gives meaning to you. It is expressed as a unique experience through and within connections to God, the Life Force, the environment, nature, other people and yourself. Spirituality and religion are not synonymous. Spirituality is a unifying force both within and beyond the self, and an aspect of humanity not subject to choice. It just exists, whereas religion is chosen. Spirituality is connected to values, but not necessarily religious values.

As you enhance your spiritual side, you begin to trust that you have the necessary resources to deal with the unexpected, and to handle anxiety-provoking situations without becoming highly anxious. You will feel your heart opening more easily to people and their concerns, and you will appreciate the interconnectedness of all life. Respecting, appreciating, and caring for the earth and all its inhabitants are elements of spirituality. Doing is the outward, visible expression of spirituality. Doing provides purpose, meaning, and strength, and spirituality is demonstrated through assisting others, being involved in environmental activities, gardening, raising children, participating in church or ritual, and visiting the sick. As your spirituality grows, you begin to experience less fear and more joy in your life, and you inspire others to do the same. You will begin to experience a sense of having everything you need in life, which will free you to get on with meeting your life purpose.

Increasing your sense of spirituality can provide the moral support, peace of mind, self-confidence, courage, hope, forgiveness, love, and faith you need to follow through on your personal anxiety-release program.

As you progress in your spirituality, you may also receive guidance. By connecting to a Higher Power or God, you can draw on this source of greater wisdom and receive answers that you might not have figured out on your own. You will begin to comprehend how all things are connected, how people and countries and even faiths are one. As you do unto the least of these, you do unto God.

You will also learn to "let go and let God." There are many situations that you cannot control, and to try to do so only increases your anxiety.

You will learn that love is stronger than fear. Most of the anxiety you feel may be due to experiencing separation, which would never occur if you felt united with others.

Ways Spirituality and Religion Can Help

Religious and spiritual ideas can help when you are highly anxious by:

- connecting you to a cause, church, or idea that distracts you from your anxiety.
- involving you by giving you a central meaning to your life.
- giving you a set of optimistic thoughts and beliefs that help you believe you will benefit from being religious or spiritual, that God or a Higher Power will help you, that devotion to these beliefs will benefit others.

The Downside of Religion and Spirituality

Although religious and spiritual thoughts and beliefs can help you, there is a downside to them.

- You can be disillusioned if you pray to God for help and it doesn't come.
- Belief in any kind of spirit, god, religion, or transcendental power can become an addiction, members of other groups

and nonbelievers can be treated with intolerance, and obsessive-compulsive behavior may result.

- Belief in religion or spiritual processes may be helpful but still leave you far from the deeper, more intensive, and enduring solutions to anxiety therapy may bring.

Whole-Brain Thinking and Spirituality

Whole-brain thinking occurs when the two cerebral hemispheres of the brain unify to create a "whole-brain thinking" pattern. Using whole-brain thinking enhances living, logic, intuition, analytical skills, mechanical reasoning, and artistic ability. It can help you expand your spiritual side.

Experimentation has shown that the two different sides, or hemispheres, of the brain are responsible for different ways of thinking. *Left-brain thinking* uses the logical, sequential, rational, analytic, objective side of your brain. It looks at parts. *Right-brain thinking* uses the intuitive, holistic, synthesizing, subjective side of your brain. It looks at wholes. Your right brain is your cradle of creativity.

Most school activity focuses on your left brain. Although left-brain thinking can be beneficial in many ways, it is this part of the brain that is responsible for worry and anxiety. By moving to whole-brain thinking you enrich brain functioning to a superior level of heightened awareness where spirituality is enhanced. *Emotional intelligence* is whole-brain thinking. It means understanding your emotions, managing them, and using them.

Here is a simple and very effective exercise to promote whole-brain functioning. Find a quiet spot, collect some paper and a pen (colored ink or felt-tip pens of various colors can add to the experience, as can listening to music that lifts your soul).

1. Think of "flow" as you handwrite the alphabet as a continuous stream (keep your pen on the paper) with your normal writing hand. A couple of times will do.

2. While thinking of "flow" again, write out the alphabet in the same fashion using your other hand.

3. Now back to your normal hand, full alphabet. Continue alternating hands and writing the alphabet until you feel the same flow using either hand (about five times with each hand). Then with your normal hand write out the alphabet twice more at the end.

You may be surprised at the changes that occur as a result, including opening you to creativity and enhanced spirituality.

Connecting with Your Higher Power (or God)

You can use prayer, meditation, or your own method of connecting with your Higher Power or God. If you like, try the exercise that follows to assist you in your quest.

1. Find a comfortable spot where you will not be interrupted.

2. Sit in a chair or lie down.

3. Breathe in relaxation and peace as a color.

4. Fill your body with the relaxing, healing color or beam of white light that dissolves your anxiety.

5. When you feel relaxed, bring to mind the person or situation that is bothering you.

6. Picture yourself handing over this problem to your Higher Power or God.

7. Say aloud or in your mind, as many times as is necessary, to let go. This may take up to an hour to connect. "I release this problem to my Higher Power [or God]," or "I ask for guidance and help with this problem."

Signs of Connection with a Higher Power

There are many happenings that can manifest in your life to let you know you have connected with your Higher Power. Some of them are:

- an intuitive recognition that you sense is true
- feelings of wonder and awe when in the presence of nature
- spontaneous healings that defy explanation
- seeing a vision of a spiritual being or presence
- an inner calmness that descends over you after a period of struggle
- feeling the support of a loving presence
- receiving the answer to an earnestly and sincerely stated prayer that serves your highest good (and doesn't interfere with anyone else's highest good)

Developing spiritually can help you see you aren't a victim with an anxiety problem but someone given an opportunity to expand who you are and what you can attain. Some new ways to understand life include:

- Your life is a training ground for something else that you cannot fully understand yet.
- Your anxiety provides a lesson; it is not a random act of fate but something that is happening for a purpose.
- Life's lessons aren't always easy, because if they were, we wouldn't grow in wisdom, compassion, and consciousness. How you respond to your anxiety may be more important than your condition. Instead of asking, "Why did this happen to me?" ask, "What can I learn from this challenge of having to deal with anxiety?"

- You have something creative to develop and offer that comes from within and has nothing to do with what your family or friends may want you to do. When you use this talent, you feel whole, complete, and fulfilled.
- Your purpose or mission can be anything, including writing, painting, speaking eloquently to groups, tending a garden in your yard, raising a healthy family, playing a musical instrument, designing clothes or buildings, or even making stuffed animals for ill adults or children.

Assessing Spirituality

Use the questions that follow to take stock and assess your spirituality.

1. Does your life have meaning?
2. Do you have a life purpose?
3. Have you set life goals for yourself?
4. Are you ready to participate in getting well?
5. Can you identify the most important thing in your life?
6. Do you know what brings you peace, joy, and satisfaction?
7. Can you be specific about what you believe in?
8. Does faith reduce your anxiety level?
9. Have you forgiven yourself for your condition?
10. Do you show love for yourself?
11. Are you close to friends or family?
12. Can you share your feelings and desires with significant others?
13. Are you able to forgive others?
14. Do you participate in any religious activities?
15. Do you participate in any activities that honor and protect the environment?
16. Do you help others in the way they wish to be helped?

17. Do you feel connected to people in other countries even if you don't know them?

18. Are you concerned about the survival of the planet?

If you can't answer yes to every one of these questions, consider putting more meaning and purpose in your life.

■ Meaning and Life Purpose

Meaning and life purpose are aspects of spirituality. If you have no meaning or purpose, it can add to your anxiety. Panic sometimes is evoked by the idea that your life has no obvious direction. Feeling trapped in an elevator, room, or house can reflect a deeper fear of being trapped in a dead-end job, relationship, or other confining situations. Phobias may reflect a deeper avoidance of taking risks that are necessary to achieve your life purpose.

Anxiety may not be fully resolved until you take responsibility to give your life a greater meaning. This could mean going to school or starting a business so you can achieve your life's purpose, or cultivating your special skills or talents.

Finding Your Life Purpose

Take time (at least a full day) to reflect on the following questions:

1. Education. Am I satisfied with the education I've obtained? If not, what education or training would I like to obtain? What is the first step toward this goal? What is the date when I will take this first step?

2. Work. Does my current work express what I really want to be doing? If it doesn't, how would I like to be making a living instead?

What is the first step toward this goal? What is the date when I will take this first step?

3. Creativity. Do I have enough creative outlets? What other areas of my life would I like to be creative in? What is the first step toward increasing my creativity? What is the date when I will take this first step?

4. Spirituality. What else would I like to do to develop my spirituality?

5. Life Dreams. What would I do with my life if I had the money and time so I could do whatever I wanted?

6. Life Accomplishments. What would I like to have accomplished by the time I reach eighty?

7. Most Important Values. Things that are most important to me in my life are:

___dedication to a social cause   ___serving others

___spiritual awareness   ___friendship

___personal growth   ___good health

___creative expression   ___peace of mind

___material success   ___happy family life

___career achievement   ___intimacy

___other (please describe):_____

8. Realizing My Values. What steps do I have to take to fully realize values that are important to me? What is the first step? On what date will I begin?

9. Undeveloped Special Talents. What steps do I need to take to develop my special talents? What is the first step? On what date will I begin?

10. My Most Important Life Purposes. What steps do I need to take to achieve my most important life purposes? What obstacles do I need to overcome to achieve my most important life purpose? What is the first step? On what date will I begin?

Visualizing Your Life Purpose

If you're still not sure what your life purpose is, try visualizing yourself achieving your life purpose. What kind of work would you be doing, and with whom? What would your living arrangements be? What would a typical workday look like?

■ Summary

Reduce anxiety by learning to enhance your relationships, life purpose, and spirituality by:

- bolstering your self-esteem
- saying no
- using assertiveness skills
- being empathic
- improving your relationships with others
- connecting with your Higher Power (or God)
- identifying and pursuing your life's purpose

PART THREE

Creating Your Anxiety Plan

11

Changes, Demands, Supports

To create Your Living Well with Anxiety plan, begin by identifying the changes, demands, and support systems that may be affecting you. The first step in this process is to fill in your Anxiety Wellness Profile. This profile will help you identify changes related to your anxiety. You will be using this profile to develop your anxiety plan, so take sufficient time to make sure you consider each item. Rate the severity of all changes you experience.

Anxiety Wellness Profile

	This affects me little, if at all.	This is a real problem, but I can function.	I can barely function with this (or thinking about this).
1. Tightness in throat	_____	_____	_____
2. Dizziness	_____	_____	_____
3. Palpitations (heart racing)	_____	_____	_____
4. Numbness	_____	_____	_____

	This affects me little, if at all.	This is a real problem, but I can function.	I can barely function with this (or thinking about this).
5. Tongue-tied	_____	_____	_____
6. Fear of losing control	_____	_____	_____
7. Fear of something bad happening	_____	_____	_____
8. Fear of a particular object or situation	_____	_____	_____
9. Repetitive thoughts or behaviors you know are irrational	_____	_____	_____
10. Stammering	_____	_____	_____
11. Discomfort in confined public situations	_____	_____	_____
12. Joint and muscle pain	_____	_____	_____
13. Fear of being home alone	_____	_____	_____
14. Feeling powerless	_____	_____	_____
15. Trembling or shaking	_____	_____	_____
16. Feeling detached or out of touch with yourself	_____	_____	_____

Changes and Demands

The changes you're undergoing are only one part of what can raise your anxiety. They use up your energy, and so do demands. The more demands you face, the less energy you have to reduce your anxiety. Check "yes" or "no" next to each change to see where you stand.

1. Being treated for a serious or chronic condition   ____ yes   ____ no

2. Raising children   ____ yes   ____ no

3. Empty-nest reaction   ___ yes   ___no

4. Change in a relationship   ___ yes   ___no

5. Change in workload   ___ yes   ___no

6. Change in job security   ___ yes   ___no

7. Dieting   ___ yes   ___no

8. Change in self-image   ___ yes   ___no

9. Loss of friend or family member   ___ yes   ___no

10. Addition to the family   ___ yes   ___no

11. Marriage   ___ yes   ___no

12. Family tensions   ___ yes   ___no

13. Separation/divorce   ___ yes   ___no

14. Moving to new residence   ___ yes   ___no

15. Vacation   ___ yes   ___no

16. Natural disaster   ___ yes   ___no

17. Remodeling   ___ yes   ___no

18. Other changes (please list):_____

19. Other demands (please list):_____

Supports

If you have sufficient supports, that can help you reduce your anxiety. Take an inventory of your support by completing the following checklist:

___ **1.** My partner listens to me and is supportive of me.

___ **2.** My partner helps out with houschold tasks.

___ **3.** My children support me.

___ **4.** My children help out around the house.

___ **5.** My parents are supportive of me.

___ **6.** One or both of my parents help out when needed.

___ **7.** I have at least one supportive friend.

___ **8.** I have at least one friend who helps out when needed.

___ **9.** I have a health-care practitioner who listens to me, explains whatever I don't understand, and is willing to consider alternative and complementary procedures.

___ **10.** I belong to a support group that provides support and understanding, information about available resources, reduced feelings of isolation, good ideas for solving common problems, hope and optimism, and a potential for new friends with common issues. The members are not overly critical or negative and do not dominate the discussion.

If you don't have enough supports, consider joining a support group, teaching your family empathy and supportive skills, finding a more supportive health practitioner (see the next chapter), or finding a new friend who's working on the same issues you are and who's supportive.

12

Finding and Working with the Right Practitioner

You may find that many of the suggestions in this book work well for you and that you don't need a health-care practitioner. Still, it's wise to at least have a practitioner available in case you need an objective reaction to your situation. Although the belief remains that people should be able to handle their own problems, in reality they can't always. Think of yourself as being mature and smart for recognizing when you need help and getting it.

> Doug used many of the methods and techniques discussed in this book and found them useful, but when he lost his job in a merger, his anxiety increased and he sought out a counselor to help him through it. Through counseling he learned how to plan out how he was going to approach job interviews, something he hadn't faced in twenty years. He started to write in a journal about his feelings, found a massage therapist, and started taking yoga classes.

As you can see from Doug's example, you may need to take a multi-faceted approach to your anxiety.

▮ Situations That Probably Require Therapy or Counseling

There are several situations that are best handled in long-term psychotherapy or counseling. One is the recall of traumatic events. Another is feeling anxious and not being able to connect current events with this feeling. A third is when feelings emerge that are too upsetting or anxiety-provoking for you to handle.

Traumatic Events

Starting to reexperience the effects of traumatic events can be anxiety-provoking, especially when you don't have an understanding of what's happening. You may have little or no recollection of the actual traumatic event, but it is affecting you nevertheless. Sometimes, if the traumatic event occurred in childhood, raising your own children can bring forth the anxiety associated with the event.

Twyla exemplifies this situation. She seemed to be perfectly fine until her daughter reached the age she was when a stranger lured her from the bus stop with candy. He drove her around and apparently didn't touch her before bringing her back to where he'd picked her up. Now Twyla experiences extreme anxiety whenever her daughter leaves the house. Until she contacted a therapist and started to talk about her life, she didn't become aware of this early experience and how it was still affecting her.

Sometimes the trauma is something that happened to you in adulthood, like rape, or observing a life-threatening occurrence. Todd, a sergeant in the army, newly returned from Iraq, and Cynthia, a woman who had been repeatedly raped by her ex-husband, exemplify this kind of situation.

The anxiety these experiences evoke can be intense and may be combined with panic. Your mind can block out the recollection to protect you. It's not a conscious choice. It's an automatic process, but it's only a temporary solution because the real cause can be set off by current events and take you by surprise.

With an experienced therapist or counselor to help you stay calm, healing is facilitated as you gradually become aware of the source of your pain. The source of your anxiety becomes clearer and clearer. Talking to a therapist about your memories, feelings, and thoughts aids in the process of recall and resolution. Once that is accomplished, you will be ready to use some of the approaches suggested in this book.

Stressful Current Events

Sometimes you may not be able to identify what is making you feel anxious. You're sure you haven't had any traumatic events in your life, but still you feel that something's wrong. You may just need somebody who can stay objective and guide you to uncover the source. This person would probably be a therapist or counselor. This person would ask you questions like, "What happened today right before you started feeling anxious?" and "What else was going on when you started to feel anxious?" As you begin to examine what happened, you'll start to make connections between your day and your feelings. Making these connections requires your willingness to start talking about what happened, to put your feelings and experiences into words, and to try to clarify connections between events in your life and your feelings.

When you first start therapy, you probably won't have any notion why you feel as anxious as you do. Just talking about stressful events enables you to begin to make connections between them and your anxiety, but it can also temporarily raise your anxiety. Sometimes this process happens quickly. Other times, it requires a lot of soul searching.

Anxiety-Provoking Feelings

You may have uncomfortable anxiety after a particular experience, even a pleasant one, and have no inkling why. Sarah is a good example of this—

Sarah was watching a movie one night and started to feel extremely anxious. She couldn't sleep that night, and the next day, upon advice of a friend, made an appointment with her friend's therapist. In just one session Sarah was able to make the connection between a tender scene in the movie between the father and daughter and her anxiety. Her father had been distant and critical, and she'd always yearned for a better relationship. When she saw the actors on the screen, it put her in touch with her conclusion that something was terribly wrong with her because her father was so unaffectionate. With support from the therapist, she was able to talk with her father and make her need for affection known. Although her father had a tough time with it, he was able to join her in a session with the therapist and tell his daughter that he did care about her, he just had a hard time showing it. Sarah's anxiety receded, and after that she had no difficulty watching films featuring affectionate fathers.

▉ Types of Practitioners

Psychotherapist is a term that applies to different types of practitioners. When choosing a psychotherapist, it's helpful to know something about the education and training of practitioners in the most common disciplines

Psychiatrists

All psychiatrists are MDs, but not all medical doctors are psychiatrists. To enter medical school an individual must complete a four-year degree such as bachelor of science (BS) or bachelor of arts (BA). Each medical school has its own specific requirements, but a strong science background is essential. Once admitted, medical students spend four years studying medicine, and the last two years usually includes practice in basic medical procedures with patients, under the supervision of other student doctors, called residents.

After graduation some medical students pursue a psychiatric residency of three to four years. After completing this residency, a physician is qualified to practice as a general adult psychiatrist (child and adolescent psychiatry requires another year or two of training). Psychiatrists take a qualifying test known as a state board exam that includes a written portion and a practical portion that tests for clinical competency with patients. To keep up with the latest information, psychiatrists must earn continuing-education credits to keep their medical license. They can obtain these credits by attending workshops, giving presentations, or writing journal articles or books.

Because of their knowledge of physiology and anatomy, they can find problems of the heart, lung, and nervous systems that may influence your anxiety. Psychiatrists are mostly concerned with prescribing and monitoring medications. Rather than conduct ongoing therapy, most psychiatrists these days work in conjunction with other mental-health professionals who provide psychotherapy.

Nurses

Most nurses complete a three-to-four-year nursing program before earning a bachelor of science in nursing (BSN) or BS in nursing. Nurses who provide psychotherapy also have a master's degree. In most states, a nurse with a master's degree is known as a Clinical

Nurse Specialist (CNS) or Psychiatric/Mental Health Nurse Practitioner (ARNP or PMHNP). Both have two or more years of education beyond the bachelor's degree and are educated to treat their clients using a more holistic method than their master's-prepared counterparts in psychology or social work (discussed below).

Most states allow CNSs and ARNPs, or PMHNPs to write prescriptions, often under the guidance of an approved supervisor with whom they have a written practice agreement.

Because of their broad education CNSs, ARNPs, and PMHNPs are also responsible for crisis intervention, client education, medication management, coordinating aspects of care, physical examinations, and mental status exams. Many CNSs perform psychotherapy, too, after having spent two years studying growth and development, theories of clinical practice, and psychiatric mental health nursing approaches and applying what they've learned with individuals, families, and groups, under supervision of more experienced nurse clinicians. Many programs require that students complete a thesis, which is a research study that focuses on a specific aspect of clinical practice. CNSs may specialize in an adult or child practice.

Once they complete their master's degrees, they continue to be supervised by a more experienced nurse psychotherapist for several thousand hours before they can take a national certifying exam to become a certified CNS, ARNP, or PMHNP. Certification is required for master's-prepared nurses who wish to practice in certain settings.

Psychologists

Psychologists complete a bachelor's degree before entering advanced training. They are educated at either the master's (MA, MS) or doctorate level (PhD, PsyD, or EdD). Some states will only license psychologists for independent practice if they are prepared at the doctorate level. Students may work in a hospital, outpatient mental health clinic, school, or any other type of facility that provides the type of work that interests them.

A psychologist with a master's degree has completed two years of advanced training in both course work and clinical work focused on personality development, abnormal psychology, tests and measurements, and theories of clinical practice. A field placement in a clinical setting is required in many programs. These students see patients under supervision and are observed by seasoned clinicians.

After graduation, a master's-prepared clinician must practice under an approved supervisor for two years, then take a national licensing exam.

Doctoral students can choose from a wide array of specialties (not all of which prepare them to be a psychotherapist), including social, industrial, school, or experimental psychology, as well as counseling and clinical practice. No matter which specialty area they choose, each student must conduct a research study, then write about it in a formal paper called a dissertation, which can take from two to seven years to complete.

After completing their degree, most schools require doctoral-level psychologists to complete 2,000 hours of work under a qualified supervisor and pass a national examination before they are licensed to practice independently.

Like psychiatrists and psychiatric mental health nurse specialists, psychologists assess, diagnose, and treat individuals seeking help. They also conduct formal personality, thought, mood, and other cognitive tests. Most states do not allow psychologists to prescribe or monitor medications.

Social Workers

Social-worker psychotherapists generally obtain a master's degree. They may have a BA in social work, but many have a degree in psychology, nursing, or education. Most advanced programs take two years and include both course work and clinical work. Specialties include clinical work and administration.

Many social-work programs consist of an ecological or systems model of treatment that focuses on an individual in the family, school, work, church, or community setting. This is similar to the advanced registered nurse practitioner model, but very different from the psychologist or psychiatrist models, which tend to focus on the individual.

Clinical social workers who become psychotherapists earn the designation Licensed Independent Clinical Social Worker (LICSW) and must complete their degree, meet all field requirements, practice for 2,000 hours under a qualified supervisor, and pass a national exam.

Clergy

Many people turn to clergy, such as their minister, pastor, or priest, for assistance with anxiety. Not all clergy are trained to treat anxiety or act as psychotherapists. Those who aren't may tend to offer you standardized advice that doesn't really relate to your specific concerns and your goals. A competent member of the clergy will refer you to a mental-health professional when the situation requires.

If you choose to work with clergy, ask about their training and credentials. Therapists hang their diplomas and licenses on the wall. Read them. Ask questions.

■ Types of Therapies

Although there are more than fifty types of therapies, this section will provide a brief overview of the more common ones.

Psychoanalysis

Psychoanalysis is based on the research and clinical experience of such major theorists as Sigmund Freud, Harry Stack Sullivan, Karen Horney, Alfred Adler, or C. G. Jung.

Although psychoanalysis acknowledges biological factors, it emphasizes internal conflicts (Freud), interpersonal issues (Sullivan), environmental and cultural factors (Horney), helplessness and inferiority complex (Alfred Adler), or spirituality, archetypes, and mythology (Jung).

To benefit from psychoanalysis, you must be able to describe and interpret your symptoms in interpersonal terms—for example, "I get anxious when my husband pressures me," or "I can't commit to a relationship with somebody because I'm afraid of getting rejected."

Psychoanalysis generally requires several sessions a week for many years. There is often little direction given by a psychoanalyst, who may say very little to you, except to make an occasional interpretation or to ask you to discuss whatever comes to mind. Relationships with important figures from your childhood are often reenacted in therapy and this *transference* becomes a focus of the work. It is called *resistance* when you don't discuss your problems in therapy.

Person-Centered Therapy

Person-centered, or client-centered, therapy was developed by Carl Rogers in the 1940s. While psychoanalysis places the analyst in the role of expert, client-centered therapy views the client as the expert and assumes you can understand yourself, and change unhealthy thoughts, feelings, and behaviors into healthier ones.

Rogers firmly believed that all people are basically trustworthy, resourceful, insightful, and capable of living effective and productive lives. Rogerian therapists provide the following characteristics during sessions, which are believed to help clients move forward in a positive manner: warmth, empathy, genuineness, and trust. Person-centered therapy focuses on the power of the therapeutic encounter. That relationship is the core of therapy. The therapist reflects back the essence of the client's feelings. For example, "I am picking up the deep sense of loss and sadness you are feeling about your husband." The person-centered therapist also opens up new areas of exploration. For example, "I'm also picking up your feeling of anger about being abandoned. Tell me more about that."

Unlike the psychoanalyst, the therapist isn't distant but appreciates your state of upset, is willing to relate to you on a more personal level, and shows unconditional positive regard for you. Psychotherapists who practice using this format do not give advice or feedback, or challenge your experience. The length of treatment varies.

If you are psychologically minded, insight-oriented, and motivated to make personal changes in your life, person-centered therapy may work well for you. If you need help with establishing goals and a treatment plan, this kind of therapy may not be for you.

Cognitive Behavioral Therapy

Cognitive behavioral therapy (CBT) was developed at the University of Pennsylvania in the 1960s by Aaron Beck, PhD. The main tenet of CBT is that thoughts determine feelings and behavior, and anxiety increases when you misinterpret situations and act on them in dysfunctional ways.

The goal of CBT is to help you test the accuracy of your perceptions and change the dysfunctional ones into more helpful ones. CBT is highly structured and directive, unlike psychoanalytic and person-centered therapies. You work with the therapist to determine your goals for treatment. You will be assigned homework between sessions to help you apply the new ways of thinking, acting, and feeling you learn in sessions. A course of CB therapy typically lasts between eight and twenty sessions.

Marriage and Family Therapy

Marriage and family therapists take a systems view of issues such as anxiety. They believe that one family member's problems are the result of unhealthy communication patterns, family roles, or family relationships within the community. Your therapist will probably ask your entire family to attend sessions, or will at least take a family view of your condition. The goal of treatment is to help your family return to a healthy state. Your therapist will be active during sessions, guiding you to help facilitate change during sessions and assigning homework between sessions to help family members practice new behaviors they need to implement.

Brief Therapy

Brief therapy is any therapy of twenty sessions or less. Any of the therapies already discussed may be brief if the therapist is trained to work in this fashion. Other names for brief therapy include "time-limited," "solution-focused," or "problem-oriented." A therapist who uses a brief-therapy approach will assess your problem, usually within the first three sessions, by asking specific questions. You will be helped to identify specific behavioral goals for treatment and be actively guided and directed toward change.

Some questions a brief therapist may ask you are:

- How would you describe yourself?
- What people or situations in your past or present do you feel angry about?
- Are you an active or passive person?
- What people or situations in your past or present do you feel guilty about?
- What is (or was) your relationship with your parents?
- What is your relationship with your brothers and sisters?
- What is (or was) your relationship to anyone else who lives (lived) in your house?
- Is your sex life satisfying?
- Are your current relationships mostly positive or mostly negative?
- Are you satisfied with your job or career?
- How would you feel if you lost the important people in your life?

Depending on how you answer, the therapist may also help you to acknowledge your feelings by helping you take a look at your defenses and the connection between your thoughts and feelings, point out mixed feelings you may have toward significant people in your life, find your buried feelings and the traps they create for you, ask if you think therapy will be helpful, place responsibility for change with you, and point out important issues for you to focus on. No advice or support is provided, but you can learn something more valuable—how to commit yourself, be clear, take action, and face painful issues.

Short-term therapists are constantly asking, "How do you feel about being here with me today?" Which helps speed up the bonding process between therapist and client. Short-term therapists will also ask questions to help you with intimacy, or with being who you really are.

These questions are intended to allow the therapist to find out your own perception of your problems, as well as to give you a sense of where your anxiety came from, how you use defenses instead of facing your problems, and some idea of what you have to do to resolve your anxiety.

■ What Qualities Make for a Good Therapist?

Researchers have studied the therapeutic process and concluded the following about therapist qualities:

- The age of your therapist is unimportant; you can do just as well with an older or a younger person.
- Try to find a therapist who is well adjusted, emotionally healthy, and with high self-esteem; working with a distressed or disturbed therapist can be harmful to you.
- You can do just as well with a male or a female therapist.

- If you're female, you'll probably fare better if your therapist holds nontraditional views of women.
- You may do better with a therapist from the same ethnic background if you're a minority client.

If you have other considerations, like the sexual orientation of a therapist or his or her views on therapy, the best thing to do is to call and ask prior to scheduling an appointment.

■ What Happens in Therapy or Counseling?

You probably have your own ideas about what happens in a psychotherapy or counseling session. No matter what kind of practitioner you choose—mental health nurse practitioner, social worker, psychologist, or psychiatrist—keep the following facts in mind. Your therapist or counselor

- will ask you to share openly your concerns, thoughts, and feelings.
- will help you take a look at your feelings and make sense of them.
- will listen objectively and help guide you toward the results you decide, not tell you what to do.
- isn't there to "change" or "fix" you, but to teach you new ways to handle your anxiety.
- is a guide to help you understand the complex nature of your anxiety and how it is related to your thoughts, beliefs, and attitudes about yourself and your world.
- may give you between-session homework assignments, such as keeping a journal, using self-rating checklists to monitor your progress, and trying out new behaviors in real-life situations.

- will use individual sessions, group-therapy sessions, or self-help books to teach you more effective ways to problem-solve and reduce your anxiety.
- can help you reduce anxiety, minimize future disasters, and develop action plans and strategies to help you grow and heal.
- cannot provide a magical solution or cure-all for your anxiety, but can be tremendously helpful during periods of high anxiety.
- will expect you to show up for scheduled sessions, pay agreed-upon professional fees, give at least twenty-four hours' notice of cancellation (except in cases of last-minute emergencies), and to pay for other missed sessions.
- may ask you to complete one or more psychological tests to help assess your needs.
- will ask you the main reason you've come for help and why you're coming at this time.
- will help you pinpoint a major focus, identify specific problems, and find out how these issues are important to you now.
- may act like a coach who can help you plan out what you want to do, practice it, get some helpful feedback, refine it, and provide the push you may need to do it in real life.
- may ask you to summarize what happened; for example, the problem, how you came to see it as understandable given your situation, that you felt okay about changing, what approaches have worked for you, how your therapist helped, and what results you got.

As the client, you may

- begin to have self-critical thoughts—for example, that you shouldn't be feeling the way you're feeling.

- feel somewhat worse in the early sessions because you've become more aware of distressing feelings.
- have a shift in attitude, from being overwhelmed to knowing you can deal with anxiety, even though you don't like the way it feels.

Try to

- not bail out during the early sessions when your anxiety may temporarily increase.
- remember that it's natural and normal to feel increased pain when you're coming to terms with important life issues, but that it's worth it because your feelings will soon make sense to you and harsh self-criticism will be reduced.

If you choose a practitioner who uses a short-term model of treatment, four key elements will be apparent:

- focus on a specific problem, not on reshaping you or your personality
- active involvement in the process that occurs between you
- emphasis on solutions, not on causes
- time-limited process

If you choose a cognitive-behavioral therapist you may be asked to

- identify the problem you want to work on and narrow it down.
- rate the target symptom or issue using a 0-to-10 rating scale.
- choose (and use) an intervention, such as thought stopping, challenging irrational beliefs, hypnotherapy, or imagery.
- rate the target symptom again.

- write down what you learned on a card or in a notebook.
- complete an assignment related to your issue between therapy sessions in order to reinforce your learning.

▮ Holistic/Complementary Therapists

Much of the daily ins and outs of anxiety involve self-care. If you face high anxiety, panic attacks, or strong phobias or obsessions, you may need a supportive practitioner. There are no anxiety specialists, although maybe there should be, but there are practitioners who can look at the broad spectrum of medical and holistic/complementary approaches.

You may start your search with your primary-care physician, or you may go directly to a therapist or counselor. Keep in mind that proper assistance may require nutrition, exercise, psychological, holistic/complementary, herbal approaches, and more. If you can find a holistically oriented general practitioner or mental-health practitioner, that's even better, because you will receive an integrated approach that includes conventional and alternative therapies, or at least referral to complementary practitioners.

I bumped into Jessica at a local library book signing. This fifty-one-year-old Sunday school teacher told me she was disappointed in her traditional physician, who gave her no time to ask questions about the medication he had prescribed for her anxiety. She asked me for some ideas. Over tea the next day we discussed her options, from types of practitioners to deciding if she wanted to switch health-care providers.

Types of Holistic/Complementary Practitioners

As a holistic/complementary practitioner myself, I believe you should have at least one holistic practitioner on your team, because anxiety responds best to a multifaceted approach. The clients I work with are grateful for my holistic approach, which helps them integrate alternative methods into their traditional approach.

Constantly changing physicians and specialists will probably not be to your advantage. Find one or more holistic/complementary practitioners who meet your criteria for service. While you're at it, check with your insurance provider to see if your visit is covered, or at least partially reimbused. It is up to you to be responsible, get educated, and learn the keys to a wellness approach to your anxiety. Some of the types of complementary practitioners available for you to consider appear below.

Acupressure Practitioners

There are various schools of acupressure, but they all involve the same pathways, or meridians, used by acupuncturists. Qi, or energy, is believed to flow along these pathways, energizing and nourishing the body, mind, and spirit. By using the hands to work these points, tensions are released and the flow of qi is enhanced.

Jin shin do practitioners teach clients how to hold specific points, and how to use breathing techniques and visualization to release distressing feelings and address neck, shoulder, back tension/pain, headache, chest problems, menstrual difficulties, pelvic tension, digestive stress, respiratory difficulties, insomnia, joint problems, creative blocks, muscle spasms, stress-related difficulties, cerebral palsy, and developmental difficulties. Because it is gentle and the recipient is clothed, jin shin do can provide safe physical touch in cases where physical or sexual abuse has occurred. For more information go to www.jinshindo.org.

Jin shin jyutsu practitioners also teach their clients self-help methods by placing the three middle fingers on "safety energy locks" in specific sequences, called "flows," to restore balance. No massage or manipulation is involved. The practitioner merely holds the lock and waits to feel the rhythmic pulsation indicating that balance has been restored. For more information, go to www.jinshin jyutsu.com. Shiatsu is the Japanese version. The whole hand is used to massage, press, and pull. In some situations, even the feet are used.

Acupuncturists

Acupuncturists insert thin, solid, usually stainless-steel needles, at precise anatomic locations—classic acupuncture points, motor points, and areas of tenderness on your body. You may wish to observe and inquire whether sterilized needles are used. An acupuncturist may manipulate these points by hand or through attached electrodes, using various wave forms and intensities of voltage. You may smell burning herbs if moxabustion is used, or feel a cupping sensation if the acupuncturist uses small jars to create a vacuum. Magnets may also be used. Acupuncturists usually learn their specialty at colleges of acupuncture and Oriental medicine (www .aaom.org), or through the American Academy of Medical Acupuncture (www.medicalacupuncture.org).

Guided Imagery Specialists

Imagery is a natural thought process that uses one or more of the five senses and is usually associated with emotions. Imagery is how your right brain conceptualizes, and it is the bridge between the conscious and subconscious mind. It is simply one way your mind thinks. Just as we all dream, we all use imagery to picture a scene in our mind's eye, or to play a pleasant memory or song back to us. For nearly 20,000 years, imagery has been an integral ingredient in healing practices, for it is the basis for the spiritual level of healing. Holistic practitioners from many disciplines practice guided imagery. To find certified practitioners, contact the Academy for Guided Imagery at 800-726-2070, or www.academyforguided imagery.com.

Herbal Practitioners

Herbology is the study of the science and artful use of healing plants, or herbs. Every culture has at some point used healing plants as the basis for its medicine. Even modern American medicine has its roots in the use of herbs. Until fifty years ago, nearly all entries in the pharmacopeias described herbs. When modern drug companies began selling synthetic medicines, the values of botanical medicines weren't preserved. Today most of the important herbal research is conducted in Europe. While traditional medicine treats specific organs (heart, mind, lungs, etc.), herbal medicine practitioners recognize that the body is an integrated system, the whole being greater than the sum of its parts. Herbalists also realize that the whole herb is greater than the sum of its parts.

Herbal preparations are only as vital as the quality of the herbs used to prepare them. Herbs are either specifics (used to treat acute conditions and used for days or weeks) or tonics (used to support and nourish body processes for months).

Since the quality and processing of herbs are hard to standardize, you should use them with caution. Consult an herbalist who has spent years getting to know the qualities, energies, and properties of herbs so that you can be matched to the herbs or combinations that best suit you. To find an herbalist, consult the American Herbalists Guild, at www.americanherbalistsguild.com.

Holistic Nurse Practitioners

Holistic nurse practitioners will not only take a complementary approach to your process, but are usually able to prescribe medications, should they be needed. They have a master's degree in nursing. More and more nursing programs are providing master's programs in holistic nursing. Many nurses with a master's degree in mental health combine a holistic approach with basic nursing knowledge. Look for a nurse practitioner who has been board certified as a holistic nurse (HNC), or, better yet, as an advanced holistic nurse (AHN-BC). These initials mean they have demonstrated their ability to work with clients in a holistic fashion. You can find certified holistic nurses by going to www.ahna.org, e-mailing info@ahna.org, or contacting the American Holistic Nurses' Association by phone at 800-278-2462.

Holistic Physicians

Like holistic nurse practitioners, holistic physicians focus on you as a whole person and on how you interact with the environment, not on illness, disease, or specific body parts. A number of medical doctors (MDs) and a larger percentage of osteopaths (DOs) practice holistic medicine and follow holistic principles. You can contact holistic physicians at the American Holistic Medical Association; for their free online directory, go to www.holisticmedicine.org.

Hypnotherapists

Hypnosis is a state of inner focus and a high degree of mental and physical relaxation during which you are more open to suggestion. Hypnotic suggestions may consist of direct commands, ideas, and mental imagery to help overcome fears and visualize the successful accomplishment of a goal. The American Society of Clinical Hypnosis provides a list of certified professional hypnotherapists at www.asch.net.

Massage Therapists

There are many kinds of massage. Neuromuscular therapy (NMT) is a form of soft-tissue massage that includes a muscle-by-muscle examination of all soft tissues that may be associated with a particular injury or pain syndrome. NMT addresses the following six factors that create or intensify pain:

1. *Ischemia*: lack of blood and oxygen caused by muscular spasm.
2. *Trigger points*: areas of increased metabolic waste deposits that excite segments of the spinal cord and cause referred pain to other parts of the body.
3. *Nerve entrapment or compression*: pressure on nerves by hard tissue (bone or disk) or soft tissue (muscle, tendon, ligament, fascia, or skin).
4. *Postural distortion*: the body is held in positions that deviate from an anatomically correct position.
5. *Poor nutrition*: either the body is getting an insufficient amount of necessary nutrients or it is getting foods that irritate the nervous system.
6. *Emotional upset*: decreased ability to withstand stress.

Swedish massage includes *effleurage* (stroking), *petrissage* (kneading, friction, or rubbing), *tapotement* (percussion), and *vibration*. Skilled practitioners work with a great sensitivity of touch rather than a mechanical routine. Smooth, long, and flowing strokes are performed with palms, finger pads, or forearms, like waves gliding and rippling over the body, bringing fresh blood, oxygen, and nutrients and taking away waste products. Short and rapid percussive movements include hacking with the outside edge of the hand, tapping with fingertips, cupping or clapping with cupped palms, pummeling with loose or tight fists, and plucking between the thumb and forefinger. Circular, linear, or transverse strokes made with the thumb, fingertips, palm, or heel of the hand provide friction that spreads muscle fibers and frees muscle from adhesions and scar tissue developed after an injury or surgery. In kneading, the practitioner lifts muscle away from bone, then squeezes, rolls, and presses it with both hands or alternates thumbs in a milking motion that flushes out fluids and metabolic byproducts. Practitioners use one hand or the fingertips to create vibration, a rapid, trembling, shaking sensation that stimulates nerves and relaxes tight muscles. The Touch Research Institute at the University of Miami School of Medicine has conducted dozens of clinical trials demonstrating that massage can facilitate growth, increase attentiveness, alleviate pain, improve immune function, and reduce stress.

Find a massage therapist through the American Massage Therapy Association (www.amtamassage.org), the Association of Bodywork and Massage Professionals (www.healthydoctors.com), or the National Association of Nurse Massage Therapists (www.nanmt.org).

Naturopathic Physicians

Naturopathy is a distinct profession of primary health care, emphasizing prevention, treatment, and optimal health using the body's self-healing processes. Doctors of Naturopathy (NDs) are general practitioners who

1. believe there is an inherent self-healing process in you that is ordered and intelligent.
2. identify and remove the underlying causes of illness rather than just eliminating or suppressing symptoms.
3. minimize the risk of harmful side effects.
4. educate clients and encourage self-responsibility for health.
5. treat the whole person.
6. assess risk factors and encourage prevention.

Naturopaths use many modalities, including nutrition, herbs, naturopathic manipulative therapy, counseling, minor surgery, homeopathy, acupuncture, and natural childbirth. Find a naturopath at the Naturopathic Medicine Network (www.pandamedicine.com.)

Reflexologists

Reflexology is based on the theory that there are reflex areas in the feet and hands that correspond to all of the glands, organs, and parts of the body. The thumbs and fingers are used to apply specific pressures to these reflex points to relieve stress, improve blood supply, relieve nerve blockages, and help the body rebalance. Clients typically express relief from tension and pain and feel a heightened sense of well-being and increased energy after a treatment. Because there are 7,200 nerve endings in each foot and each has extensive interconnections through the spinal cord and brain, all areas of the body can be treated by working with the feet.

Some form of reflexology existed in ancient Egypt at least as far back as 2300 B.C., but it was an American, Dr. William H. Fitzgerald, who discovered the Chinese method of zone therapy now known as reflexology. To find out more about the procedure and to find reflexology practitioners, go to www.reflexology.org.

Relaxation Therapists

Progressive muscle relaxation (PMR) training is a simple and effective form of treatment for helping people learn to relax. The procedure can be used as a primary treatment to complement medical care. It was developed by Dr. Edmund Jacobson in 1929. Jacobson discovered that by using a prescribed system of tensing and releasing of muscles, deeper levels of relaxation could be reached than by sitting quietly and trying to relax. He based his treatment on the theory that the body responds to anxiety and stress by producing muscle tension, which creates anxiety. He believed that deep muscle relaxation was incompatible with anxiety. The two could not exist at the same time.

In PMR you are taught to tense and release muscles or muscle groups (for example, your leg) while being helped to focus on the difference between tension and relaxation. This prepares you to more easily relax your muscles at will. You may even be asked to repeat a calming phrase, such as, "I am relaxing." PMR can usually be learned in one to three weeks if practiced as recommended. There are no cautions, although if the tensing of muscles is overdone, cramping can result. If you're taking a tranquilizer, PMR may enable you to decrease your dosage. To find a therapist, go to the Directory of Approved Natural Health Practitioners at www.nchm .net/DANHP/relax.htm.

Tai Chi Instructors

Tai chi is a series of slow, gentle movements designed to enhance mind and body function. It is usually practiced outdoors and is a kind of moving meditation. Each move has a symbolic meaning. Many Chinese practice it every morning, and it is believed to be the most widely practiced exercise in the world. Because of its gentle nature, it is appropriate for any age. Research studies show the movements improve awareness of different body parts and have positive effects on the heart and blood vessels, the bones, the muscles, and even the nervous system. Its tranquil nature reduces stress and stress-related conditions. To find a tai chi teacher, go to www.thetaichisite.com/tai-203.htm.

Yoga Teachers

Yoga in Sanskrit means "union of the different aspects of a person." *Hatha* yoga is a way of controlling the mind through mastery of the body, using postures and breathing conducive to meditation and bodily control. Yogic body postures make up the majority of hatha yoga, which has been found to help relieve high blood pressure, depression, and osteoporosis and to aid in menopausal discomfort. Each posture was inspired by the natural surroundings of ancient India, and they are named for them—for example, the tree pose, the cobra pose, etc. When the posture is said aloud, *asana* is often added, which means calm, steady state or seat. Asana also implies that each posture is a prelude to the ultimate goal of hatha yoga, being comfortable and healthy.

A qualified instructor is recommended, especially if health issues need to be addressed. Go to the website of the American Yoga Association (www.americanyogaassociation.org) or the International Association of Yoga Therapists (www.iayt.org).

Choosing a Practitioner

You probably spend a lot of time finding a good accountant, dentist, insurance company, baby sitter, or auto mechanic. Make sure you make at least as much effort finding your health-care practitioner. Prior to looking for a practitioner, decide on the qualities that are important to you.

Gender

Consider whether you'd rather work with a male or female practitioner. Female physicians tend to spend more time with their patients than their male counterparts, according to a study conducted at the University of California and published in the *Journal of the American Medical Women's Association*. The results provide evidence that female physicians spend a significantly greater proportion of visits on preventive services and counseling than male physicians do, and that male physicians devote more time to technical practice behaviors and discussions of substance abuse.

A review of studies done between 1967 and 2001 concluded that medical visits with female physicians averaged two minutes (10 percent) longer than those with male physicians. Female physicians engaged in significantly more communication that could be considered patient-centered. They engaged in more active partnership behaviors, positive talk, psychosocial counseling, psychosocial questioning, and emotionally focused talk. Patients of female physicians spoke more overall, disclosed more biomedical and psychosocial information, and made more positive statements to their physicians than the patients of male physicians. Only in the field of obstetrics and gynecology did male physicians demonstrate higher levels of emotionally focused talk than their female colleagues.

Race

There hasn't been a lot of research done on race and its effect on how you're treated, but one study showed that African-American consumers who visit physicians of the same race rate their medical visits as more satisfying and participatory than those who see physicians of other races. Race-concordant visits are longer and characterized by more positive patient feeling. The association between race concordance and higher ratings of care is independent of patient-centered communication, suggesting that other factors, such as patient and physician attitudes, may be at work.

Another study examining referrals to specialists found that white physicians were more likely than black physicians to rate previous experience with the specialist and board certification to be of major importance. White physicians were somewhat less likely than black physicians to rate patient convenience to be of major importance.

Physician Practice Style

Style of physician-patient interaction has been shown to have an impact on health outcome. Researchers at Case Western Reserve University observed 2,881 patients visiting 138 family physicians for outpatient care in 84 community family practice offices in northeastern Ohio. Physicians with person-focused style rated highest on four of five measures of quality of the physician-patient relationship and patient satisfaction. Physicians with a high-control style were lowest or next to lowest on outcomes. Physicians with a person-focused style granted the longest visits, while high-control physicians held the shortest visits, a difference of two minutes per visit on average. The differences could not be explained away by patient and physician age and gender.

Physician Communication Style

Physician communication style is important to your health. Studies have shown that when patients are informed and involved in decision making, they are more apt to follow medical recommendations and to carry out more health-related behavior changes. A major study reported in the *Journal of the American Board of Family Practice* provided a review of studies done from 1975 to 2000 that evaluated the office interactions between primary-care physicians and patients, using neutral observers who coded what they saw or heard. The researchers concluded that physicians should focus on patient satisfaction, understanding, empathy, courtesy, friendliness, reassurance, support, and encouragement, on answering questions, giving explanations, and reinforcing good feelings about patient actions. Physicians ought to listen, provide health education, summarize patient statements, talk on the patient's level, and clarify what they mean. Patient satisfaction after a visit was decreased by excessive biomedical questioning, as well as by instances of doctors interrupting patients when they were speaking. Physicians ought to avoid being unduly dominant, angry, nervous, and directive. Several researchers also emphasized the importance of patients being involved in decisions about their care.

A study conducted at the Johns Hopkins University School of Hygiene and Public Health examined communication patterns of primary-care physicians. The researchers found five distinct communication patterns:

1. narrowly biomedical, characterized by closed-ended medical questions and biomedical talk (observed in 32 percent of the visits)

2. expanded biomedical, similar to the restricted pattern but with moderate levels of psychosocial discussion (observed in 33 percent of the visits)
3. biopsychosocial, reflecting a balance of psychosocial and biomedical topics (20 percent)
4. psychosocial, characterized by psychosocial exchange (8 percent)
5. consumerist, characterized primarily by patient questions and physician information giving (8 percent)

Biomedically focused visits were observed more often with sicker, older, and lower-income patients attended by younger male physicians. Physician satisfaction was lowest in the narrowly biomedical pattern and highest in the consumerist pattern, while patient satisfaction was highest in the psychosocial pattern.

Referral to Specialists

In most cases, your primary-care physician will refer you to a specialist. What do primary-care physicians consider to be important criteria in the specialists to whom they're referring you? One study found that the most important were medical skill, appointment timeliness, insurance coverage, the doctor's own previous experience with the specialist, quality of specialist communication, specialist efforts to return patient to primary physician for care, and the likelihood of good patient-specialist rapport.

Similarity to Other Practitioners

A study of family physicians (FPs) and naturopathic practitioners (NPs) found that patients perceived no difference in patient-centered care between FPs and NPs. The same was true of nurse practitioners and physicians. In a study conducted at the University of Texas at Arlington, clinic patients perceived no difference in health and satisfaction with care whether the care was given by a nurse practitioner or a primary-care physician.

Consumer Beliefs

Effective communication is a critical component of quality health care. A study at Texas A&M University examined the relative control exerted over the practitioner-consumer relationship by practitioners and consumers. Patients who preferred shared control were more active, expressing more opinions, concerns, and questions than consumers oriented toward physician control. Physicians used more partnership building with male patients. Approximately 14 percent of patient participation was prompted by physician partnership building, and 33 percent of physician partnership building was in response to active patient participation. In other words, if you ask more questions and express more opinions and concerns, you're more apt to evoke partnership building in your practitioner.

Cost/Coverage

Many holistic and complementary practitioners are not covered by health-maintenance organizations (HMOs) or insurance plans. You may have to decide whether you're willing to pay additional money or a copayment to work with one.

Credentials

Many practitioners display their credentials conspicuously on their office walls, but you have a right to ask practitioners where they went to school and what specific things they studied, as well as what continuing education courses they took that could make them especially helpful to you.

Experience/Success

In addition to education, practitioners' experience may be important to you. Feel free to ask how many highly anxious people they've worked with and their success rate.

Certification

Being board certified means that a practitioner has had clinical experience and passed a competency exam in a particular area of expertise. If this is important to you, ask practitioners you're considering whether they are board certified. Although board certification doesn't guarantee that a practitioner can help you, it is one measure you can use to evaluate their preparation.

Disciplinary Action

You may want to know if a practitioner has had any disciplinary actions taken against him or her. In some states you can find this information about physicians and nurse practitioners on the state's health department website. Do an Internet search using terms such as "Department of Health, Florida" (or whatever state you live in).

Flexible Hours

If you work or have other time constraints, a practitioner's office hours may be important to you. Call prior to making an appointment to find out hours of practice and if home visits are possible.

References

You may want to talk to other consumers who've used the practitioner's services. Ask for references, then call or e-mail them to ask whatever you'd like to know about the practitioner.

Screening Practitioner Candidates

Once you've decided on the type(s) of practitioner(s) with whom you want to work, ask around. Friends, family, and other health-care professionals can provide the names of practitioners they recommend. Ask them what they like and don't like about a practitioner and what their experiences have been with that individual.

When you've narrowed down your choices to a short list, start calling the practitioners, speak with the office manager or practitioner and ask the following questions. Add any others you may have.

- Are you accepting new clients?
- Do I need a referral?
- What are your hours?
- Am I apt to get switched to another practitioner without advance notice?
- Who would I be likely to be switched to?
- How long am I likely to be kept waiting when I have an appointment?
- What fee do you charge per session?
- What insurance, Medicaid, and Medicare coverage do you accept?
- What copayments do you charge?
- What deductibles are due at my first visit?
- Is full payment required at the time of the appointment or can I work out a payment schedule?
- How long do I have to wait to get an appointment?
- Do you charge for missed appointments?
- How quickly do you return phone calls?
- Do you give advice over the phone or by e-mail?
- Do you provide sessions at home or at work?
- Do you provide handouts for treatment options and home-work, and do you involve me in treatment decisions?

- Do you perform lab work in your own office or send it out to an independent laboratory?
- Can you provide references from consumers who have used your services?

If you can't get answers to these questions and any other information you require to make an informed decision, move on to another practitioner. A relationship with a health-care practitioner who refuses to respect your right to be involved in decisions about your care isn't in your best interest.

When you've eliminated most practitioners based on this process, you may want to visit a practitioner's office and/or set up an appointment with a practitioner to learn more. Be aware that you may be charged for this visit. Many of your questions (maybe most) can be answered by observing the practitioner and staff in action. The information you gather will help you decide which health-care practitioner best suits your needs. Here are some other things to ask before settling on a practitioner:

- Can you give me samples of your diagnostic, evaluation, health education, and prevention forms?
- Who are the alternative/complementary practitioners you use for referrals?
- What side effects does this medication (treatment) have?
- Do you have any literature about this medication (treatment) I can have?
- Do I get to undress and dress in private?
- What treatment and payment options do I have?
- What will you teach me about the medicines or treatments you prescribe?
- What kind of input do I have into decisions about my care?

- How comfortable are you answering my questions about health care?
- How interested are you in my opinions and feelings?

Also observe: Do staff members . . .

- treat you with respect?
- gossip or share private information about other clients?

Does the practitioner . . .

- keep you waiting for your appointment?
- take time to learn about you, your background, and your lifestyle?
- patiently explain all treatments/medications and their pros and cons?
- answer all your questions to your satisfaction?
- admit or show through facial expression that he or she isn't comfortable answering your questions?
- act irritated or impatient or ignore your requests for explanations?
- talk about research findings you found in this book, in the media, or online?
- accept written materials about you or research findings you bring in and promise to read them?
- dismiss all information but his or hers as quackery or uninformed?

When you return from your first visit, reevaluate your selection. If you're not comfortable, motivated, and feel you've not been treated well, visit another practitioner on your list.

Communicating with Your Practitioner

You are the one most interested in reducing your anxiety and the best person to keep track of all your health-care records. Ask for copies, not a handwritten summary, of all notes and tests (laboratory and otherwise) and provide a stamped self-addressed envelope so the office manager knows you're serious. Keep all information, organized by date, in a loose-leaf notebook. Use dividers to separate the notebook by lab work, consultation, X-ray reports, and so on, for easy reference.

Keep track of dates of visits to practitioners, as well as of injections, vaccinations, special treatments, diagnostic procedures, dosage levels of medication (and when begun and ended), blood-test results, diagnosed diseases, surgeries, hospitalizations, major emotional and physical stresses, and your own progress notes (life changes, how they affect your anxiety, nutrition/stress management/herbal and other actions taken to reduce anxiety, which ones work and which ones don't).

Preparing for Appointments

Time is money for practitioners, so if you go to your health-care appointments well organized, you're more likely to be treated with respect. To have a successful visit:

- Fax ahead or mail in advance any research articles or information you want your practitioner to read.
- Bring a friend or family member who is assertive and who can speak up for you in a diplomatic way in the event you are highly anxious. Even if you're not anxious, bringing someone along for support is a good idea and provides a second set of ears and eyes. If your practitioner gives you a hard time about your having someone along, hold your line. You're paying the bill and should be able to decide who you want to bring into the examining or treatment

room with you. As long as the person who accompanies
you doesn't have an active communicable infection and re-
frains from touching anything in the room, there shouldn't
be a problem. Even better, bring a health-care professional
with you. Be sure you share your agenda with your friend
or provide a copy of your list so you both know the points
you want to cover. That person can also take notes or help
you re-create what happened after the appointment ends.

- Bring a copy of the names and dosages of all medications,
  supplements, and herbs you are taking, as well as any other
  complementary treatment you're using.
- Treat each appointment as if it were an important business
  meeting, which it is. The business is your health, so take it
  seriously. Remember: the practitioner works for you. Dress
  for success by wearing a suit. Avoid apologizing when you
  ask for information and explanations. You deserve to know
  the rationale behind any treatment or medication that is
  prescribed.
- Write down your main concerns and present them in their
  order of importance to you.
- Take notes on your practitioner's comments whenever you
  can. Between you and your friend, you should have all important points covered.
- Ask *all* your questions. Whenever the practitioner says
  something you don't understand, say, "I'm not sure I understand what you mean. Would you please repeat it in less
  technical language?"

As you gather information about practitioners, rate each item according to its importance to you, then compare practitioners, choosing the one(s) who most closely resemble your required qualities.

Practitioner Checklist

Practitioner Qualities	Important	Not Important
1. Is the same gender as I am.	_____	_____
2. Is the same race as I am.	_____	_____
3. Shares decision making with me.	_____	_____
4. Shows interest in my opinions and feelings.	_____	_____
5. Is supportive.	_____	_____
6. Is respectful.	_____	_____
7. Explains rationale for tests and treatments.	_____	_____
8. Explains how referral decisions are made.	_____	_____
9. Cost for treatment is covered by my insurance.	_____	_____
10. Credentials are adequate to provide good treatment.	_____	_____
11. Has had experience and success with similar clients.	_____	_____
12. Is board certified in a relevant specialty.	_____	_____
13. Has no disciplinary action on record.	_____	_____
14. Has flexible hours of treatment.	_____	_____
15. Provides client references.	_____	_____
16. Is accepting new clients.	_____	_____
17. Will take me on without a referral.	_____	_____
18. Sees me within five minutes of my appointment time.	_____	_____
19. Requires copayment.	_____	_____
20. Allows me to work out a payment schedule.	_____	_____
21. Never switches me to another practitioner without advance notice.	_____	_____
22. Fits me in for an appointment.	_____	_____

Practitioner Qualities	Important	Not Important
23. Doesn't charge for missed appointments when notified within twenty-four hours.	_____	_____
24. Returns my phone calls promptly.	_____	_____
25. Is willing to give advice over the phone or by e-mail.	_____	_____
26. Provides handouts about medication and treatment options and their side effects.	_____	_____
27. Sends out blood and other test samples to an independent lab.	_____	_____
28. Refers to alternative/complementary practitioners.	_____	_____
29. Staff is professional and does not gossip about or share information about other clients in my presence.	_____	_____
30. Takes time to learn about me, my background, and lifestyle.	_____	_____
31. Patiently explains all treatments/medications and their pros and cons.	_____	_____
32. Answers all my questions to my satisfaction.	_____	_____
33. Takes whatever written materials about me or research findings I provide and discusses them with me.	_____	_____

Remember that your health practitioner needs to be your partner in wellness decisions. Find a compassionate, informed person who will work with you, not dictate to you, so that together you can find the right solutions for you.

13

Putting It All Together: Your Anxiety Success Plan

Now that you have read this far, you have all the information you need to put together your personal anxiety success plan. One thing to always keep in mind is that anxiety, like other emotions, is often created by your attitude. If you enter a situation with the attitude that you aren't competent and don't have the skills you need, you've already defeated yourself. Staying positive is crucial to success. A negative outlook puts up a barrier between you and reality. So whatever you choose to do, make sure you stay positive. You can do it!

The best way to reduce your anxiety and keep it manageable is to use the information in this book to develop your own personalized wellness plan. If you invest the time and effort required to make a plan and follow it through, you will be way ahead of the game and well on your way to living well with anxiety.

▉ When You Get Bogged Down

To notice a change in your level of anxiety, you must actually do the exercises suggested in this book—answer the questions, set your goals, evaluate your progress, and write down your thoughts and feelings. If you find yourself losing interest, ask and answer the following questions:

- Is it really important to me to reduce my anxiety?
- What would I rather be doing than working to reduce my anxiety?
- Is the thing I'd rather be doing more important in the long run than reducing my anxiety?
- Can I reschedule so I can do both?
- If I don't follow through with this project now, when exactly will I?
- What would I have to give up if I reduced my anxiety?
- What would I have to confront if I reduced my anxiety?

▉ Identifying Your Excuses

Change doesn't always come easily. Are you making excuses for why you're not following the suggestions in this book? Identify which of the following excuses you use:

- I'm too busy.
- I'm too tired.
- I'll do it tomorrow.
- I'm bored.
- I'm feeling better, so why bother?
- It probably won't work anyway.

Many of these excuses have a bit of truth in them. You may be tired or bored, but that alone isn't the total answer. Maybe your answer is, "I'm tired and bored, and I'd rather spend my time sleeping."

Whether you choose to follow the suggestions in this book or not, the important factor is that you take responsibility for your actions. Don't pretend you're a victim of circumstances. You're in charge of you.

Hint: the excuses you tell yourself are probably the same ones you've used to perpetuate old habits in the past. These excuses are based on faulty beliefs—for example, the belief that you can't change, or that you'll never be able to master the activities, or even that you don't deserve to feel better.

It may surprise you to learn that you may be attached to your anxiety. It's familiar, after all. And it may serve an important function in your life. Your anxiety may relieve you of social obligations you find unpleasant without disappointing others. This is called *secondary gain*. How can anyone be disappointed when you're in such distress?

To determine if you're receiving secondary gain, keep a log of when your anxiety occurs, and what activities, or potential activities, surround it. You may think you're anxious in all social settings but find you're only anxious when you have to speak to a stranger or to a group of people.

Secondary gain often dates back to a specific event. Remember when your anxiety began to skyrocket. You may find you share your tendency for high anxiety with a family member. For example, your mother and you may both believe that new situations are scary. With this kind of anticipation hounding you, any new situation brings fear with it.

If you can't remember or decide what belief system you share with a family member, consider consulting a professional therapist or counselor to help you identify patterns and beliefs.

Persist in your efforts to manage your anxiety. You can alter your anxiety by changing the structure of your thoughts. Stick with it!

▌ A Contract Could Help

It may not be enough to make promises to yourself because eventually you may return to old patterns. This can happen if the commitments you make to yourself aren't as important in your estimation as the ones you make to others. Maybe you believe it's okay to disappoint yourself because no one cares or even notices.

Making a written contract with a trusted friend or colleague can help if you have a tendency not to follow through on things. Make sure you choose someone you don't want to let down, someone who knows and cares about you.

If a friend's opinion doesn't motivate you sufficiently, write in a penalty clause, such as donating to a cause you hate the most, or weeding the garden, or some other task you don't enjoy. If your penalty clause includes money, have your friend hold the check, only to mail it in if you fail to fulfill your contract.

Official Contract

I will reduce my anxiety by using the following techniques:

1. _____

2. _____

3. _____

I have sworn to _____ (your friend's name) to practice the three techniques listed above _____ times a day/week for _____ days/weeks.

I promise to evaluate my improvement at the end of this period, and I will notify the above-mentioned person if I fail to uphold this contract.

_____   _____

Your Signature   Date

Official Contract

I will periodically check with _____ (your name) to remind her/him that progress on reducing anxiety is important to me.

_____   _____

Support Person's Signature   Date

If I fail to uphold this contract, I promise to _____.

If my penalty includes money, _____ (support person) will hold the check until notified and will then mail it to the address on the envelope.

Every anxiety journey is unique. The key is to find the right approach for you.

▌ Attitude Is Important

Viewing anxiety as a normal human process is a step in the right direction. But it's not all roses, even when you find the right mix of self-care to help you feel energetic.

Whether or not you're able to reduce your anxiety as much as you'd like, try to remain positive about the process. The more you invest yourself in dealing with your anxiety in a constructive way, the more likely you are to have a positive experience.

▌ Coordinate Your Wellness Team

Once you've chosen your wellness team, it will be up to you to coordinate their efforts. At least you've chosen them, so you know they'll be on your side and supportive of your objectives.

At certain times, you might have to be assertive, encouraging practitioners to talk to each other so your treatment is coordinated. You can help by . . .

- giving each practitioner a current list of your drugs, nutritional supplements, herbs, and complementary and self-care measures.
- asking each practitioner to provide a written summary of your work together.
- encouraging practitioners to speak with each other if there is any disagreement among them, and include you in the discussion, perhaps via a conference call.

If one or more of your practitioners refuses to collaborate, this is a red flag that it's time to replace them with more cooperative team members.

When you have a working team, be sure to put their names and specialties in your wellness plan notebook, along with their phone numbers, cell numbers, fax numbers, and other identifying information.

■ Choosing Your Self-Care Options

Let's take a look at some examples of other individuals who have experienced anxiety and learned to reduce it to a manageable state.

Audrey, a fifty-two-year-old accountant, called me because she didn't want to continue taking medications that she knew had many unwanted side effects and which weren't helping her to leave the house. She'd been suffering from high anxiety ever since her father died. That's when she started smoking again. About a year later, her husband left her, claiming her obsessive behavior and inability to leave the house drove him away. She suffered from tightness in her throat, palpitations, fear of losing control, repetitive thoughts and behaviors she knew were irrational, and embarrassment. Using the information in chapters 5 through 10, I coached her to develop her own anxiety wellness plan. She agreed not to write down any action she didn't think she would follow. That way we built in more chances for success.

Check out Audrey's plan. You'll notice anxiety symptoms run down the left side of the form and the types of approaches run across the top of the form. Audrey only filled in the parts that related to her changes and only used the suggestions from chapters 5 through 10 that appealed to her. She wrote N/A (not applicable) in the areas that didn't apply.

Audrey's Living Well with Anxiety Plan

Anxiety Symptoms	Nutrition	Herbs	Environment	Exercise	Stress Reduction/ Healing	Relationships/ Spirituality
Tightness in Throat	Avoid eating dry foods like crackers, chips, bread, popcorn. Eat more juicy fruit, soups, vegetable juices.	Drink 1–3 cups chamomile tea a day.	Follow stop-smoking plan.	Take a yoga class on TV or purchase video or DVD.	Use this affirmation: "My throat is relaxed and calm."	Take an online assertiveness class.
Palpitations	Avoid caffeine, chocolate, simple sugars, sweets, and salt. Eat more fish, legumes, veggies, whole grains. Use rosemary when cooking.	Peppermint tea after meals. Take nutmeg capsules for sleep.	Avoid news and violent shows or movies.	Work in my garden daily. Cook with iron pots.	Affirmation: "My heart beats slow and regular."	Develop a desensitization hierarchy for events that make my heart race.

Anxiety Symptoms	Nutrition	Herbs	Environment	Exercise	Stress Reduction/ Healing	Relationships/ Spirituality
Fear of Losing Control	Take B-complex 50 mg with meals. Eat more salmon, almonds, oats, broccoli, prunes, cabbage, turnips.	Take bupleurum.	Use time-management skills.	Do laps in my pool.	Affirmation: "I am in control of my process." Counting meditation.	Let go and let God.
Repetitive Thoughts	Eat more egg yolks, lima beans, pecans, sardines, pumpkin seeds, sunflower seeds.	Take ashwaganda.	Use lavender in diffuser.	Walking. Meditation.	Affirmation: "My mind is clear; all is well." Thought stopping. Refute irrational ideas.	Challenge my shoulds.
Repetitive Behaviors	Eat more apples, green leafy vegetables, apricots, avocados, figs, blackstrap molasses, brown rice, figs, soy.		Listen to Beethoven.		Affirmation: "I am in control of my body."	Erase faulty tapes.

Anxiety Symptoms	Nutrition	Herbs	Environment	Exercise	Stress Reduction/ Healing	Relationships/ Spirituality
Embarrassment			Sit in the sun.	Dance in my room.	Breathe in violet color when overexcited.	Practice taking criticism.
Stammering	N/A					
Discomfort in Confined Places	N/A					
Fear of Being Home Alone	Take 500 mg vitamin C and an additional B-complex.	Try biota seeds	Use ylang-ylang in diffuser.		Use coping thoughts: "I can do this." Use imagery to prepare for being home alone.	Call a meeting for family support. Try connecting with a Higher Power.
Feeling Powerless	N/A					
Numbness	N/A					
Trembling or Shaking	N/A					
Feeling Detached	N/A					

Ted, a thirty-year-old father of triplets and a licensed physical therapist, complained of anxiety symptoms different from Audrey's, which is not unusual. Anxiety affects different people in different ways. Ted suffered from intense anxiety whenever he had to speak in front of a group and often stammered. After he lost his job working for an HMO, he began to get anxious in confined places, which made it difficult for him to go for job interviews and sometimes gave him an unreal feeling of being detached. By then he also complained of feeling powerless and numb and reported that he sometimes trembled when he thought about what had happened to him. As we worked together, he revealed flashbacks and nightmares about his stint in the army. Using information found in chapters 5 through 10, I helped him construct his Living Well with Anxiety Plan.

Ted's Living Well with Anxiety Plan

Anxiety Symptoms	Nutrition	Herbs	Environment	Exercise	Stress Reduction/ Healing	Relationships/ Spirituality
Tightness in Throat	N/A					
Palpitations	N/A					
Fear of Losing Control	N/A					
Repetitive Thoughts	N/A					
Repetitive Behaviors	N/A					
Embarrassment	N/A					
Stammering	Eat more fish, almonds, oats, broccoli, turnips, green leafy vegetables, cabbage, prunes.	Sip chamomile tea at meetings/ interviews.	Use lavender in diffuser at meetings.	Massage throat before interviews or meetings.	Use coping thoughts: "I can stay relaxed and focused." Use role-play.	Challenge my shoulds. Practice active listening. Practice taking criticism.

Anxiety Symptoms	Nutrition	Herbs	Environment	Exercise	Stress Reduction/ Healing	Relationships/ Spirituality
Discomfort in Confined Places	Eat a mainly vegetarian diet. Eat brown rice, figs, soy, apples, avocados.	Take bupleurum.	Play soothing music through earphones.	Do weight lifting.	Count breaths. Use imagery to picture the room looking less confining. Play relaxation tape through earphones.	Erase faulty tapes. Connect with Higher Power and ask for help.
Fear of Being Home Alone	N/A					
Feeling Powerless	Eat more flaxseed muffins, Brazil nuts. Drink green tea.		Reward self with power clothes and accessories.	Weight lift to power up.	Use autogenics to relax. Affirmations: "I am strong. I am powerful."	Find a like-minded support group.
Numbness	Eat less meat and sugar. Stop skipping meals. Eat more salmon, oats, prunes, green leafy vegetables, almonds, broccoli, turnips, cabbage.	Try a cup of blue vervain.	Take a sun break, not a coffee break.	Take tai chi to get in touch with my body.	Play relaxation tape.	Draw to get in touch with my feelings.

Anxiety Symptoms	Nutrition	Herbs	Environment	Exercise	Stress Reduction/ Healing	Relationships/ Spirituality
Trembling or Shaking	Eliminate caffeine, sugar. Eat more apples, greens, avocados, apricots, figs, blackstrap molasses, brown rice, soy.	Valerian to relax muscles.	Carry a sweater or wear a vest.	Do yoga to relax. Rub webbing between thumb and index finger.	Use coping thoughts: "I refuse to let anything upset me." Affirmation: "I can stay calm." Picture self calm and relaxed.	
Feeling Detached	Take B-complex. Drink green tea.	Sip peppermint tea.	Follow time-management script to stay focused.	Swim to feel safe.	Do thought stopping to stay focused.	Remind myself of my rights.

The blank form for your anxiety wellness plan appears on the next page. Copy it for your own use. (A downloadable version of this form is also available online at http://HolisticHealth.bellaonline.com.)

Your Living Well with Anxiety Plan

Anxiety Symptoms	Nutrition	Herbs	Environment	Exercise	Stress Reduction/ Healing	Relationships/ Spirituality
Tightness in Throat						
Dizziness						
Palpitations						
Tongue-tied						
Fear of Losing Control						

Anxiety Symptoms	Nutrition	Herbs	Environment	Exercise	Stress Reduction/ Healing	Relationships/ Spirituality
Fear of Something Bad Happening						
Fear of a Particular Object or Situation						
Repetitive Thoughts						
Repetitive Behaviors						
Embarrass-ment						

Anxiety Symptoms	Nutrition	Herbs	Environment	Exercise	Stress Reduction/ Healing	Relationships/ Spirituality
Stammering						
Discomfort in Confined Public Situations						
Fear of Being Home Alone						
Feeling Powerless						
Numbness						

Anxiety Symptoms	Nutrition	Herbs	Environment	Exercise	Stress Reduction/ Healing	Relationships/ Spirituality
Trembling or Shaking						
Feeling Detached or Out of Touch						

I hope the information, ideas, and resources in this book will inspire you and guide you toward finding your optimal wellness team and creating your own anxiety wellness plan. Write to me with your experiences, questions, ideas, comments on the book, or to share your own story. You can contact me by e-mail or sign up for my *Holistic Health Newsletter* at http://HolisticHealth.bellaonline.com.

Best wishes on your journey. May it be the best time of your life!

RESOURCES

I've included resources that can help you find more detailed information on specific topics that are crucial to healing your anxiety condition. If you want ongoing information on self-care approaches to anxiety, please visit my website at http://HolisticHealth.bellaonline.com. You'll find updates on topics discussed in this book.

Websites and E-mail Addresses

About Our Kids.org
www.aboutourkids.org/articles/guidetopsychmeds.html
"Guide to Psychiatric Medications for Children and Adolescents," available from New York University's Child Study Center. Covers types of medications, what they are prescribed for, and their side effects for antipsychotics, antidepressants, stimulants, and SSRIs.

Alexander Technique
www.alexandertechnique.com/teacher/northamerica/
www.alexandertechnique.com/teacher/northamerica/#Canada
Advocates of this technique believe that both physical and mental-health problems are partly caused by the incorrect use of the body over many years, often since childhood. They believe that if people habitually adopt an incorrect posture, with tensed muscles, humped backs, crossed legs, and jutting chins, the nervous system and the muscles cannot function properly. The Alexander Technique retrains the patient in the correct use of the body, so that a conscious awareness of correct posture and body alignment is developed. The process involves relearning many activities that are taken for

granted, such as sitting, standing, lying down, getting up, and walking. One of the main aims is to "free the neck" through an awareness of the tension in the neck and shoulders and the use of special techniques to release this tension.

American Academy of Child and Adolescent Psychiatry
www.aacap.org

See the AACAP's award-winning fact sheets written for the help of children and their families. Especially useful are "Psychiatric medication for children," and "Questions to ask about psychiatric medications for children and adolescents."

American Academy of Environmental Medicine
www.aaem.com

This is the U.S. organization of clinical ecologists. Provides support groups, conferences, materials, and information on the effects of environment on illness.

American Society of Clinical Hypnosis
www.asch.net

Anxiety Disorders Association of America
www.adaa.org
self-help@adaa.org

The Anxiety Disorders Association of America (ADAA) is a nonprofit, charitable organization that promotes public awareness about anxiety disorders, stimulates research and development of effective treatments, and offers assistance to sufferers and their families to find available specialists and treatment programs. You can search for a therapist or support group (or even start one!) by city or zip code. Also offered is information about the variety of mental health practitioners available and a series of questions to ask providers prior to beginning treatment with them.

Anxiety Network International

www.anxietynetwork.com

ascaz@concentric.net

The Anxiety Network is an international outreach to educate and inform the general public about anxiety disorders, and to educate and support individuals with anxiety disorders. The website provides information, support, and therapy for the most prevalent anxiety disorders: social anxiety (social phobia), panic/agoraphobia, and generalized anxiety. Contact: Dr. Thomas Richards, by filling out the e-mail form on the website.

Association for Applied Psychophysiology and Biofeedback

www.aapb.org

The website provides articles on biofeedback, diseases which conditions are most treatable by this method, and includes biofeedback news, a bulletin board, and books and pamphlets both for the general public and for professionals.

Awareness Foundation for OCD and Related Disorders

www.ocdawareness.com

Awareness9@aol.com

This foundation combines the expertise and experience of dynamic workshop speakers with the emotional impact of film to increase understanding of obsessive-compulsive disorder and related disorders. Contact: James Callner, M.A., 435 Alberto Way, Suite 3, Los Gatos, CA 95032.

Biofeedback Society of America

Maintains a list of certified biofeedback practitioners. Contact them at 10200 44th Avenue, Suite 304, Wheat Ridge, CO 80033-2840, 800-477-8892.

Center for Anxiety and Stress Treatment

www.stressrelease.com

health@stressrelease.com

The Center for Anxiety and Stress Treatment has a variety of resources that aid in stress reduction, including books, audiotape-based anxiety-reduction programs, and workshops. Their mission is to provide resources that can help consumers manage and regain their lives. Contact: Shirly Babior, LCSW, 4225 Executive Square, Suite 1110, La Jolla, CA 92037.

Center for Mindfulness in Medicine, Health Care & Society
www.umassmed.edu/cfm/tapes

For guided-meditation tapes by Jon Kabat-Zinn, go to their website and click on "Mindfulness Meditation Practice Tapes."

At the University of Massachusetts Medical Center, patients are encouraged to listen to soothing music and to perform relaxation exercises and meditation. This innovative program was developed by Jon Kabat-Zinn, director of the stress reduction and relaxation program, and harpist Georgia Kelly. It offers a safe, natural alternative to tranquilizers and other mood-altering drugs.

CHAANGE
www.chaange.com
info@chaange.com

The Center for Health, Anxiety and Agoraphobia for New Growth Experiences (CHAANGE) provides a four-month program based on cognitive (thought-based), behavioral, and goal-oriented theories. The first phase of the program defines anxiety conditions, tells you how and why they likely developed for you, and describes what happens in your body when you experience them. The second phase teaches you how to relax your body to counteract the tension that anxiety produces. You will be given relaxation exercises, which we encourage you to practice until they become automatic. The third and fourth phases will teach you thinking, attitude, belief, and behavior skills that will change your current nonproductive patterns and, in effect, turn your life around. When you enroll in the program, you will be provided with the following materials over the course of the sixteen weekly sessions: workbook, weekly interactive audio cassette tapes, two books, homework materials, magazine and journal reprints, review sheets, and a three-ring binder notebook. You are also provided with a free subscription to the monthly newsletter, *exCHAANGE,* and periodic evaluation forms to monitor your progress. You can also work face to face with a CHAANGEaffiliated therapist on a weekly basis. These are professional, licensed, independent practitioners from the fields of psychology, medicine, counseling, social work, and other related disciplines, who have been thoroughly trained in the CHAANGE methodology. You have the option of working with CHAANGE by yourself at home. You can arrange weekly shipments of the program sessions from our national headquarters. CHAANGE en Español and LifeSkills for anxious children are also available, along with many self-help books and tapes produced by CHAANGE.

FDA Drug Safety Initiative
www.fda.gov/cder/index.html
This Food and Drug Administration site provides information about drug safety.

Feldenkrais Guild
www.feldenkrais.com
toll-free number: 866-333-6248
The Feldenkrais Method is for anyone who wants to reconnect with their natural abilities to move, think, and feel, reduce pain, focus attention, and be able to participate in once-enjoyed activities. Whether you want to be more comfortable sitting at your computer, playing with your children and grandchildren, or performing a favorite pastime, these gentle lessons can improve your overall well-being. FEFNA, 3611 SW Hood Ave., Suite 100, Portland, OR 97239.

Freedom from Fear Friends Club
www.freedomfromfear.org/search
As part of the Freedom From Fear's Friends Club you can be connected with a pen pal (or as many as you wish). Membership also includes the following: newsletters featuring the latest in the treatment of psychiatric illnesses, access to their Referral Network, an invitation to educational seminars, an invitation to join International Pen Pal Network, and help in organizing support groups.

Greenhome Environmental Superstore

www.greenhome.com

info@greenhome.com

A complete environmental online store including bath, bedding, furniture, home furnishings, home improvement, housekeeping, kids, kitchen, lighting, office, personal accessories, pest control, pets, water, yard and garden, testing materials (water, pesticides, electromagnetic fields).

Mental Health Net

www.mentalhelp.net

info@centersite.net

Mental Help Net is a comprehensive source of online mental-health information, news, and resources. The MHN website discusses disorders such as depression, anxiety, and substance abuse, and also makes professional journals and self-help magazines available online. Contact: 570 Metro Place North, Dublin, OH 43017.

National Anxiety Foundation

www.lexington-on-line.com/naf.html

A volunteer nonprofit entity that aims to educate the public and professionals about anxiety disorders through print and electronic media. Contact: 3135 Custer Drive, Lexington, KY 40517-4001.

National Mental Health Consumers' Self-Help Clearinghouse

www.mhselfhelp.org

info@mhselfhelp.org

This consumer-run national technical assistance center promotes consumer/survivor participation in planning, providing, and evaluating mental-health and community-support services. It provides technical assistance and information to consumer's providers interested in developing self-help services and advocating to make traditional services more consumer oriented. Contact: 1211 Chestnut Street, Suite 1207, Philadelphia, PA 19107.

Obsessive-Compulsive Foundation

www.ocfoundation.org

info@ocfoundation.org

The Obsessive-Compulsive Foundation (OCF), with more than 10,000 members, is an international nonprofit organization composed of people with obsessive-compulsive disorder (OCD) and related disorders, their families, friends, and professionals. Founded by a group of individuals with OCD in 1986, the mission of the OCF is to educate the public and professionals about OCD and related disorders; to provide assistance to individuals with OCD and related disorders, as well as to their families and friends; and to support research into the causes and effective treatments of OCD and related disorders.

OCF resources and activities include: bimonthly newsletters designed to provide people with OCD, their families, and friends with the very latest in information on research, resources, and recovery; annual three-day membership conferences; and the Behavior Therapy Institute (BTI), designed to train mental-health professionals in the latest techniques to treat OCD. Organizes and promotes OCD-related support groups and OCF affiliates around the country and abroad. Distributes a wide range of articles, pamphlets, books, audio- and videotapes about OCD and related disorders, many of which are funded and produced by OCF. Maintains a Treatment Providers List of professionals throughout the country who treat individuals with OCD and related disorders (available upon request from the Obsessive-Compulsive Foundation, Inc., 676 State Street, New Haven, CT 06511; phone 203-401-2070; fax: 203-401-2076; e-mail: info@ocfoundation.org).

The OCD Resource Center of South Florida

www.ocdhope.com

ocdhope@bellsouth.net

Disseminates information about new developments in the treatment of obsessive-compulsive disorder (OCD). Estimates that three to five million adults and half a million children nationwide suffer from this disabling disorder. The website describes available serivces for children and adults, including assessment and evaluation, medication, individual cognitive-behavior therapy, and group and family therapy. Contact: 3475 Sheridan Street, Suite 310, Hollywood, FL 33021.

Open Doors Institute

www.opendoorsinstitute.com
info@opendoorsinstitute.com

Based on techniques developed by Dr. Lynne Freeman, this organization provides cognitive-behavioral therapy, psychiatric evaluation, phone sessions, and a network of providers.

Recovery, Inc.

www.recovery-inc.com
inquiries@recover-inc.com

This international community mental-health organization offers a self-help method of training: a system of techniques for controlling temperamental behavior and changing attitudes toward nervous symptoms, anxiety, depression, anger, and fear.

Relaxation Techniques

Numerous clinics and hospitals around the country have integrated relaxation techniques into their care. To learn more about relaxation techniques and to locate facilities that include them, go to www.umassmed .edu/cfm/mbsr.

Social Phobics Anonymous

www.healsocialanxiety.com
healsocialanxiety@hotmail.com

Offers a free twelve-step recovery program for individuals who have an unreasonable fear of social situations. Free face-to-face support groups are offered in Boulder, Colorado, at the First Presbyterian Church. Telephone conference support groups are accessible by anyone anywhere who possesses a phone. Call 303-404-3747 to get access code for conference group.

UCLA Center for Mental Health in Schools

http://smhp.psych.ucla.edu

smhp@ucla.edu

The following documents can be downloaded at no cost from the website: "Affect and Mood Problems Related to School Aged Youth," "Anxiety, Fears, Phobias, and Related Problems: Intervention and Resources for School Aged Youth," and "Common Psychosocial Problems of School Aged Youth: Developmental Variations, Problems, Disorders and Perspectives for Prevention and Treatment," among others.

Audiocassettes and CDs for Relaxation

Letting Go of Stress, by Emmett Miller, M.D., available from Source, P.O. Box W, Stanford, CA 94305, or call 800-52-TAPES

Relaxation Training Program, by Thomas Budzynski, Ph.D., available from Guilford Publications, 72 Spring Street, New York, NY 10012, or call 800-365-7006 (outside Manhattan) or 212-431-9800 (in NYC).

Driving Far from Home, by Edmund J. Bourne and Jerry Landis. One 120-minute cassette. To order, call New Harbinger Publications at 800-748-6273.

Music for the Mozart Effect: Volume II, Heal the Body; Music for Rest and Relaxation, 800-427-7680.

Books

An End to Panic: Breakthrough Techniques for Overcoming Panic Disorder by Elke Zuercher-White, Ph.D. Oakland, California: New Harbinger Publications, Inc., 1998.

This state-of-the-art program covers breathing retraining, taking charge of fear-fueling thoughts, overcoming the fear of physical symptoms, coping with phobic situations, avoiding relapse, and living life in the here and now.

The Anxiety and Phobia Workbook by Edmund J. Bourne, Ph.D. Oakland, California: New Harbinger Publications, Inc., 1995.

This practical and comprehensive guide can help you if you struggle with panic attacks, agoraphobia, social fears, generalized anxiety, obsessive-compulsive behaviors, or other anxiety disorders. Provides step-by-step guidelines, questionnaires, and exercises to help you learn skills and make lifestyle changes needed to achieve a full and lasting recovery. Can be used as an adjunct to therapy.

The Body Image Workbook: An 8-Step Program for Learning to Like Your Looks by Thomas F. Cash, Ph.D. Oakland, California: New Harbinger Publications, Inc., 1997.

If the way you think you look contributes to your anxiety, this may be the book for you. The program presented in this book has been clinically tested with others just like you, and shows you exactly how to transform a negative body image into a more pleasurable, affirming relationship with your appearance.

Children Changed by Trauma: A Healing Guide by Debra Whiting Alexander, Ph.D. Oakland, California: New Harbinger Publications, Inc., 1999.

Shows parents and others what to do to help a child that has witnessed a traumatic event. It provides advice on how to help children cope with emotions, learn to talk about what happened, and begin to feel safe again.

Consumer's Guide to Psychiatric Drugs by John D. Preston, Psy.D., John H. O'Neal, M.D., and Mary C. Talaga, R.Ph., M.A. Oakland, California: New Harbinger Publications, Inc., 1999.

You'll find a complete explanation of how each drug works and detailed information about treatment for anxiety and sleep disorders, as well as depression and a wide range of other conditions.

The Daily Relaxer by Matthew McKay, Ph.D., and Patrick Fanning. Oakland, California: New Harbinger Publications, Inc., 1997.

Distills the best of the best to bring together the most effective and popular techniques for learning how to relax. These simple, tension-relieving exercises can be learned in less than ten minutes and can help you achieve positive results right away.

Dying of Embarrassment: Help for Social Anxiety and Social Phobia by Barbara G. Markway, Ph.D., *et al*. Oakland, California: New Harbinger Publications, Inc., 1992.

This book provides clear and supportive ways to assess your fears, improve or develop new social skills, and change self-defeating thinking patterns.

Family Guide to Emotional Wellness by Patrick Fanning and Matthew McKay, Ph.D. Oakland, California: New Harbinger Publications, Inc., 2000.

This book is a compilation of the two author-publishers' work over the past twenty years and covers nearly 200 self-help titles in psychology and health. It includes information on how to get along in a family, with kids, if you have addictions (eating, alcohol, drugs, smoking, gambling, or Internet), how to cope with physical problems, bad moods, and painful feelings (there are six chapters related to anxiety), how and when to get help, and how to optimize your life with relaxation, meditation, visualization, and dream analysis.

Heal Your Body A–Z by Louise L. Hay. Carlsbad, California: Hay House, Inc., 1998.

Discusses the mental causes for physical illness and the way to overcome them, including the probable cause of anxiety and panic from a metaphysical viewpoint. Also includes new thought patterns (affirmations) to use to reduce anxiety.

Helping Your Anxious Child: A Step-by-Step Guide for Parents, by Ronald M. Rapee, Ph.D., *et al.* Oakland, California: New Harbinger Publications, Inc., 2000.

I Can't Get Over It: A Handbook for Trauma Survivors by Aphrodite Matsakis, Ph.D. Oakland, California: New Harbinger Publications, Inc., 1996.

This groundbreaking work can help you cope with traumatic memories and emotions, identify triggers that reactivate traumatic anxiety, relieve secondary wounding, and gain a sense of empowerment and hope.

Illuminata, by Marianne Williamson. New York: Random House, 1994.

An outstanding collection of prayers and thoughts for connecting with your Higher Power or God.

The Relaxation and Stress Reduction Workbook by Martha Davis, Ph.D., Elizabeth Robbins Eshelman, M.S.W., and Matthew McKay, Ph.D. Oakland, California: New Harbinger Publications, 2000.

This book offers simple, concise, step-by-step directions for mastery of breathing, progressive relaxation, meditation, self-hypnosis, visualization, refuting irrational ideas, thought stopping, worry control, coping skills, exercise, nutrition, time management, assertiveness, job-stress management, and quick relaxers.

The Relaxation Response by Herbert Benson, M.D., and Miriam Z. Klipper. New York: HarperCollins, 2000.

This book was first published in 1975 and is a classic. Using a mind/body approach to stress reduction, Dr. Benson shows that relaxation techniques such as meditation can lower blood pressure and reduce heart disease. It demystifies the mantra meditation and explains how to use it.

Self-Esteem by Matthew McKay, Ph.D., and Patrick Fanning. Oakland, California: New Harbinger Publications, Inc., 2000.

This is the most comprehensive guide on the subject. It contains proven cognitive techniques for assessing, improving, and maintaining high self-esteem by talking back to the critical voice inside you. Also included in this third edition is a chapter on changing core beliefs that hinder you from setting and achieving goals in your life. It covers the importance of goal setting in maintaining high self-esteem, and discusses how to set realistic goals and break them into manageable steps; also covered are the blocks to achieving goals and how to overcome them.

The Stop Smoking Workbook: Your Guide to Healthy Quitting by Lori Stevic-Rust, Ph.D., and Anita Maximin, Psy.D. Oakland, California: New Harbinger Publications, Inc., 1996.

Smoking can create more anxiety for you. It's time to quit. This workbook gives you the tools to change. Guided by challenging exercises, you start by learning how to assess your smoking habits. Soon you'll learn other coping techniques, find the best strategies for making it through the first weeks, and discover how to minimize your chances of smoking again.

Think Like a Shrink: Solve Your Problems Yourself with Short-Term Therapy Techniques by Christ Zois, M.D. New York: Time Warner, 1992.

Dr. Zois, a leader in the short-term psychotherapy movement and a highly respected clinician at two leading medical schools, tells you how to achieve major breakthroughs and bring lasting changes that help you to identify your buried feelings and how they trap you. You will also learn how to isolate your defenses against knowing yourself and overcome them, eliminate negative behaviors that sabotage you, develop successful intimate relationships, and stop being a victim.

Thoughts and Feelings: Taking Control of Your Moods and Your Life by Matthew McKay, Ph.D., Martha Davis, Ph.D., and Patrick Fanning. Oakland, California: New Harbinger Publications, Inc., 1998.

This complete and useful guide provides cognitive behavioral techniques for taking control of your moods. It includes twelve step-by-step, research-based protocols that combine the most effective techniques for treating problems ranging from panic disorder to obsessional thinking.

The Three Minute Meditator by David Harp, with Nina Feldman, Ph.D. Oakland, California: New Harbinger Publications, Inc., 1996.

If you don't think you have time to meditate, try this down-to-earth introduction to the basics of using meditation to cope with stress and anxiety in your daily life. You can find self-acceptance and inner peace.

Understanding Your Child's Sexual Behavior: What's Natural and Healthy by Toni Cavanagh Johnson, Ph.D., Oakland, California: New Harbinger Publications, Inc., 1999.

This book can put your mind at ease if you're a parent. It shows you how to differentiate between worrisome and natural or healthy behavior and can free you from misconceptions about sexual abuse.

Visualization for Change by Patrick Fanning. Oakland, California: New Harbinger Publications, Inc., 1994.

This classic includes applications for weight control, stopping smoking, stress and anxiety reduction, self-esteem, insomnia, shyness, creativity, problem solving, and more.

When Once Is Not Enough: Help for Obsessive Compulsives by Gail Steketee, Ph.D., and Kerrin White, M.D. Oakland, California: New Harbinger Publications, Inc., 1990.

How to recognize and confront fears, use simple exercises to block rituals, keep going with positive coping strategies, and handle complications and relapses.

Working It Out: Using Exercise in Psychotherapy, by K. F. Hays. Washington, D.C.: American Psychological Association, 1999.

Recommends that practitioners prescribe exercise to aid the recovery from mental health conditions. The author provides detailed information regarding the effects of exercise on well-being and the use of exercise regimens custom-tailored to client needs and abilities, and also addresses ethical issues relevant to exercise.

The Worry Control Workbook by Mary Ellen Copeland, M.S., M.A. Oakland, California: New Harbinger Publications, 1998.

Based on an extensive research study, the author has built a practical self-help program that shares the experiences of those who have developed ways to overcome chronic worry. Combines easy-to-follow strategies and techniques with a step-by-step, interactive format. Helps identify the place worry plays in your life, as well as areas where specific types of worry are likely to reoccur, and teaches you how to develop new skills for dealing with them.

Your Drug May Be Your Problem: How and Why to Stop Taking Psychiatric Medications
by Peter R. Breggin, M.D., and David Cohen, Ph.D. Reading, Massachusetts: Perseus Books, 1999.

This book is the only volume that provides an up-to-date, uncensored description of the dangers involved in taking every kind of psychiatric medication, including Prozac, Effexor, Zoloft, Paxil, Luvox, Elavil, Pamelor,

Xanax, Valium, Klonopin, Ativan, Dalmane, lithium, Depakote, Haldol, Risperdal, Navane, Clozaril, Zyprexa, ritalin, dexedrine, and Adderall. The book is the first and only book to explain how to safely stop taking them. It can help you and your doctor make a plan to safely withdraw you from psychiatric drugs and will help you maintain control over your own psychiatric treatment.

REFERENCES

Chapter 1 Anxiety: Causes and Effects

Clark, C.C. "Anxiety in the nurse-patient relationship." In *Nursing Concepts and Processes*. Albany, New York: Delmar Publishers, 1977.

———. *Wellness Practitioner*. New York: Springer Publishing Company, Inc., 1996.

Johnson, J.G., P. Cohen, and D.S. Pine. "Association between cigarette smoking and anxiety disorders during adolescence and early adulthood." *Journal of the American Medical Association* 284:2348–51, 2000.

Sherman, C. "Alcohol complicates, compromises anxiety treatment." *Clinical Psychiatry News*, October, 2004, p. 26.

Sullivan, H.S. "The meaning of anxiety in psychiatry and life." Washington, D.C.: William Alanson White Psychiatric Foundation, 1948.

———. *The Interpersonal Theory of Psychiatry*. New York: W.W. Norton & Company, 1951.

Zolot, J.S., and D. Sofer. "Anxiety is increasing in children." *American Journal of Nursing* 101 (3):18, 2001.

Chapter 2 Self-Diagnosing Your Anxiety

Bourne, E.J. *The Anxiety & Phobia Workbook*. Oakland, California: New Harbinger Publications, Inc., 1995.

Clark, C.C. "Anxiety in the nurse-patient relationship." In *Nursing Concepts and Processes*. Albany, New York: Delmar Publishers, 1977.

———. *Wellness Practitioner*. New York: Springer Publishing Company, Inc., 1996.

Chapter 3 Types of Anxiety Disorders

American Psychological Association. "Anxiety Disorders: The role of psychotherapy in effective treatment." Practice Directorate, APA, Washington, D.C.: APA, 1998. (http://helping.apa.org/therapy/anxiety.html)

Deci, P.A., R.B. Lydiard, A.B. Santos, and G.W. Arana. "Oral contraceptives and panic disorder." *Journal of Clinical Psychiatry* 53(5):163–65, 1992.

Diagnostic and Statistical Manual of Mental Disorders. Fourth Edition. Washington, D.C.: American Psychiatric Association, 1994.

Finn, R. "Study shows high rate of psychiatric polypharmacy." *Clinical Psychiatric News.* January 5, 2005, p. 50.

———. "Emotional disclosure is key to PTSD," *Clinical Psychiatry News.* January 2005.

Jancin, B. "CBT improves Post-CABG depression in women." *Clinical Psychiatry News.* July 2005, p. 57.

Laraia, M. "Panic." *Advance for Nurse Practitioners.* December 1995, pp. 24–29.

Storz, D.R. "Getting a grip on anxiety." *The Clinical Advisor,* March 1999, pp. 17–26.

Chapter 4: Anxiety, Your Brain, and Medication

"Benzodiazepines." www.usdoj.gov/ndic/pubs07/717/odd.htm: Accessed 7/20/05.

Breggin, P.R., and D. Cohen. *Your Drug May Be Your Problem, How and Why to Stop Taking Psychiatric Medications.* New York: Perseus, 1999.

Crowley, M. "Better than Prozac: An evening with Samuel Barondes. www.nyas.org.

Mindell, E., and V. Hopkins. *Prescription Alternatives.* New Canaan, Connecticut: Keats Publishing, Inc., 1998.

Longo, L.P., and B. Johnson. "Addiction: Part 1. Benzodiazepines—Side effects, abuse risk and alternatives. www.aafp.or/afp/200000401/2121.htm.

Munoz, R.A. "The truth about the drug companies." www.eclinicalpsychiatrynews.com, accessed December 2004.

"Prescription drugs kill more Floridians than illegal drugs." *St. Petersburg Times,* June 8, 2002.

Preston, J.D., J.H. O'Neal, and M. Talaga. *Consumer's Guide to Psychiatric Drugs.* Oakland, California: New Harbinger Publications, Inc., 1998.

Rosack, J. "Research reveals more about alcoholism's complex action on brain." *Psychiatric News,* volume 37, number 18, 2002, p. 21.

Schneider, M.E. "New APA president vows to restore specialty's credibility." *Clinical Psychiatry News.* July 2005, p. 64.

Stahl, S.M. "Why drugs and hormones may interact in psychiatric disorders." www.psychiatrist.com/pcc.brainstorm/br6204.htm.

Stevens, L. "Psychiatric Drugs: Cure or quackery?" www.antipsychiatry.org.

Wolf, B.C., *et al.* "Alphazolan-related deaths in Palm Beach County." *American Journal of Forensic Medicine and Pathology,* 26(1):24–27, 2005.

"Xanax." www.homedrugtestingKit.com/xanax.html: accessed 7/19/05.

Chapter 5 Nutrition

Balch, J.F. and P.A. Balch. *Prescription for Nutritional Healing.* Garden City Park, New York: Avery Publishing Group, 1997.

Bell, R.A. "An epidemiologic review of dietary intake studies among American Indians and Alaska Natives, implications for heart disease and cancer risk." *Annals of Epidemiology* 7(4):229–40, 1997.

Bjelland, I., *et al.* "Folate, vitamin B_{12}, homocysteine, and the MTHFR 677C-T polymorphism in anxiety and depression: the Hordaland Homocysteine Study." *Archives of General Psychiatry* 60(6):618–26, 2003.

Botella, P., and A. Parra. "Coffee increases state anxiety in males but not females." *Human Psychoparmacology* 18(2):141–43, 2003.

Brody, S. "High-dose ascorbic acid increases intercourse frequency and improves mood: a randomized controlled clinical trial." *Biological Psychiatry* 52(4):371–74, 2002.

Calder, P.C. "N-3 polyunsaturated fatty acids and immune cell function," *Advanced Enzyme Regulation* 37: 197–237, 1997.

Carroll, D., *et al.* "The effects of an oral multivitamin combination with calcium, magnesium, and zinc on psychological well-being in healthy young male volunteers: a double-blind placebo-controlled trial." *Psychopharmacology* 150(2):220–25, 2000.

Cartwright, M., *et al.* "Stress and dietary practices in adolescents." *Health Psychology* 22(4):362–69, 2003.

Colantuoni, C., *et al.* "Evidence that intermittent, excessive sugar intake causes endogenous opioid dependence." *Obesity Research* 10(6):478–88, 2002.

Covington, M.B. "Omega-3 fatty acids." *American Family Physician* 70(1):133–40, 2004.

Goldman, R., R. Klatz, and L. Berger. *Brain Fitness, Anti-Aging Strategies for Achieving Super Mind Power.* New York: Doubleday, 1999.

"The good fats—are you getting enough?" *Better Nutrition.* August 2000, pp. 42–47.

Grimaldi, B.L. "The central role of magnesium deficiency in Tourette's syndrome: casual relationships between magnesium deficiency, altered biochemical pathways and symptoms relating to Tourette's syndrome and several reported comorbid conditions." *Medical Hypotheses* 58(1):47–60, 2002.

Jones, A.Y., E. Dean, and S.K. Lo. "Interrelationships between anxiety, lifestyle self-reports and fitness in a sample of Hong Kong University students." *Stress* 5(1):65–71, 2002.

Mark, V.H., and J.P. Mark. *Brain Power, a Neurosurgeon's Complete Program to Maintain and Enhance Brain Fitness Throughout Your Life.* Boston: Houghton-Mifflin, 1989.

Menotti, A. "Food intake patterns and 25-year mortality from coronary heart disease: cross cultural correlations in the seven countries' study," *European Journal of Epidemiology* 15(6):507–25, 1999.

Nutt, D.J., C.J. Bell, and A.L. Malizia. "Brain mechanisms of social anxiety disorder." *Journal of Clinical Psychiatry* 59(Supplement 17):4–11, 1998.

Rodriguez, J.J., J.R. Rodriguez, and M.J. Gonzalez. "Indicators of anxiety and depression in subjects with different kinds of diet: vegetarians and omnivores." *Biological Association of Medicine* 90(4–6):58–68, 1998.

Rountree, R. "Anxiety: Natural choice is L-theanine." www.letsliveonline.com, April 2002.

Smriga, M., *et al.* "Lysine fortification reduces anxiety and lessens stress in family members in economically weak communities in Northwest Syria." *Proceedings of the National Academy of Sciences* 101(22):8285–88, 2004.

Sonee, M., *et al.* "The soy isoflavone, genistein, protects human cortical neuronal cells from oxidative stress." *Neurotoxicology* 25(5):885–91.

Song, C., *et al.* "Effects of dietary n-3 or n-6 fatty acids on interleukin-1beta-induced anxiety, stress, and inflammatory responses in rats." *Journal of Lipid Research* 44(10):1984–91, 2003.

Wild, R., ed. *The Complete Book of Natural and Medicinal Cures.* Emmaus, Pennsylvania: Rodale Press, 1994.

Chapter 6 Herbs

Angelo, M., and A.L. Miller. "Nature's pharmacy: Anxiety." www.lets liveonline.com, June 2001, p. 24.

Balch, J.F. and P.A. Balch. *Prescription for Nutritional Healing.* Garden City Park, New York: Avery Publishing Group, 1997.

Castleman, M. *The Healing Herbs.* Emmaus, Pennsylvania: Rodale, 1991.

Connor, K.M., J.R., Davidson, and L.E. Churchill. "Adverse-effect profile of kava." *CNS Spectrum* 6(10):848–53, 2001.

Geier, F.P., and T. Konstantinowicz. "Kava treatment in patients with anxiety." *Phytotherapy Research* 18(4), 297–300, 2004.

Hoffman, D. *Herbs to Relieve Stress.* New Canaan, Connecticut: Keats Publishing, Inc., 1996.

Keville, K. *Herbs for Health and Healing.* Emmaus, Pennsylvania: Rodale, 1996.

Landis, R. *Herbal Defense.* New York: Warner, 1997.

Martin, C. *Earthmagic: Finding and Using Medicinal Herbs.* Woodstock, Vermont: Countryman Press, 1991.

Mowrey, B. *The Scientific Validation of Herbal Medicine.* New Canaan, Connecticut: Keats Publishing, Inc., 1986.

———. *New Generation Herbal Medicine.* New Canaan, Connecticut: Keats Publishing, Inc., 1990.

———. *Herbal Tonic Therapies.* New Canaan, Connecticut: Keats Publishing, Inc., 1993.

"Natural anxiolytics—kava and L.72 anti-anxiety formula." *American Journal of Natural Medicine* 1(2):10–14, 1994.

Teeguarden, R. *Radiant Health: The Ancient Wisdom of the Chinese Tonic Herbs*. New York: Warner, 1998.

Chapter 7 Environmental Changes

Fanning, P., and M. McKay. "Alcohol and Drugs." In *Family Guide to Emotional Wellness*. Oakland, California: New Harbinger Publications, Inc.

Isensee, B., *et al*. "Smoking increases risk of panic: findings from a prospective community study." *Archives of General Psychiatry* 60(7): 692–700, 2003.

Johnson, J.G., P. Cohen, and D.S. Pine. "Anxiety disorders preceded by years of heavy smoking." *Clinician Reviews* 11(2):55, 59, 2001.

Righi, E., *et al*. "Air quality and well-being perception in subjects attending university libraries in Modena." *Science of the Total Environment* 286(1–3):41–50, 2002.

Sherman, C. "Alcohol complicates, compromises anxiety treatment." *Clinical Psychiatry News* October 2004. p. 26.

Williams, D.G. "Safe 'shuteye'—natural remedies for insomnia." *Alternatives* 6(4):25–31, 1995.

Chapter 8 Exercise

Beckfield, D.F. *Master Your Panic and Take Back Your Life! Twelve Treatment Sessions to Overcome High Anxiety*. Atascadero, California: Impact Publishers, Inc., 2001.

Boenisch, E., and C.M. Haney. *The Stress Owner's Manual*. Atascadero, California: Impact Publishers, Inc., 2001.

Jones, A.Y., E. Dean, and S.K. Lo. "Interrelationships between anxiety, lifestyle self-reports and fitness in a sample of Hong Kong University students." *Stress* 5(1):65–71, 2002.

Kugler, J., H. Seelbach, and G.M. Kruskemper. "Effects of rehabilitation exercise programmes on anxiety and depression in coronary patients: a meta-analysis." *British Journal of Clinical Psychology* 33 (pt. 3):410, 1994.

Leste, A., and J. Rust. "Effects of dance on anxiety." *Perceptual Motor Skills* 58(3): 767–72, 1984.

Mock, V., *et al.* "Effects of exercise on fatigue, physical functioning, and emotional distress during radiation therapy for breast cancer." *Oncology Nursing Forum.* 24(6):991–100, 1997.

O'Connor, P.J., *et al.* "State anxiety and ambulatory blood pressure following resistance exercise in females." *Medical Science in Sports and Exercise* 25(4):516–21, 1993.

Pierce, E.F., and D.W. Pate. "Mood alterations in older adults following acute exercise." *Perceptual Motor Skills* 79 (part 1):191–94, 1994.

Raglin, J.S., P.E. Turner, and F. Eksten. "State anxiety and blood pressure following 30 minutes of leg ergometry or weight training." *Medical Science in Sports and Exercise* 25(9):1044–48, 1993.

Rejeski, W.J., *et al.* "Acute exercise: buffering psychosocial stress responses in women. *Health Psychology* 11(6): 355–62, 1992.

Vedral, J.L. *Definition, Shape Without Bulk in 15 Minutes a Day!* New York: Warner Books, 1995.

Chapter 9 Other Anxiety-Reducing and Healing Measures

"Anxiety." *Update on Human Behavior* 11(2A):1–4.

Ashton, C., Jr., *et al.* "Self-hypnosis reduces anxiety following coronary artery bypass surgery. A prospective randomized trial." *Journal of Cardiovascular Surgery* 38(1):69–75, 1997.

Barnason, S., L. Zimmerman, and J. Nieveen. "The effects of music interventions on anxiety in the patient after coronary artery bypass grafting." *Heart and Lung* 24(2):124–32, 1995.

Beck, A.T., and G. Emergy. *Cognitive therapy of anxiety and phobic disorders.* Philadelphia: Center for Cognitive Therapy, 1979.

———. *Anxiety Disorders and Phobias.* New York: Basic Books, 1985.

Beck. A.T., *et al.* "A crossover study of focused cognitive therapy of panic disorder. *American Journal of Psychiatry* 149, 778–83, 1992.

———. "Beyond belief: A theory of modes, personality, and psychopathology." In Paul M. Salkovskis, ed. *Frontiers of Cognitive Therapy.* New York: Guilford Press, pp. 1–25, 1996.

Beck, J.G., *et al.* "Comparison of cognitive therapy and relaxation training for panic disorder." *Journal of Consulting and Clinical Psychology* 62(4):819–26, 1994.

Beddows, J. "Alleviating preoperative anxiety in patients: a study. *Nursing Standards* 11(37): 35–38,1997.

Benson, H. *The Relaxation Response.* New York: William Morrow and Company, 2000.

"Benzodiazepines," www.usdoj.gov/ndic/pubs07/717/odd.htm, accessed 7/16/05.

Bonn, J.A., C.P. Readhead, and B.H. Timmons. "Enhanced adaptive behavioural response in agoraphobic patients pretreated with breathing training." *Lancet* 2(8404):655–59, 1984.

Borysenko, J. *Minding the Body, Mending the Mind.* Reading, Massachusetts: Addison-Wesley, 1987.

Brown, G.K., *et al.* "A comparison of focused and standard cognitive therapy for panic disorder." *Journal of Anxiety Disorders* 11(3):329–45, 1997.

Caruba, A. "Worry your way to success: Ten secrets to successful problem solving plus where to find help." Maplewood, New Jersey: The National Anxiety Center, 1992.

Clark, C.C. "Post traumatic stress disorder, Part 2—Interventions." *The Nursing Spectrum* March 25, pp. 12–14, 1996.

———. *Holistic Assertiveness Skills for Nurses.* New York: Springer Publishing Company, Inc., 2003.

———. *Group Leadership Skills.* New York: Springer Publishing Company, Inc., 2003.

———. "Some quick ways you can reduce stress." *The Wellness E-Newsletter* 1(1):1–6, 2004.

G.A. Clum, and R. Surls. "A meta-analysis of treatments for panic disorder." *Journal of Consulting and Clinical Psychology* 61(2):317–26, 1993.

Collinge, W. "Chinese Medicine: The Cosmic Symphony." *The American Holistic Health Association Complete Guide to Alternative Medicine.* New York: Warner Books, 1987.

————. "Ayurveda: The Wisdom of the Ancients." In *The American Holistic Health Association Complete Guide to Alternative Medicine*. New York: Warner Books, 1987.

Crisp, T. *Liberating the Body*. London: Aquarian Press, 1992.

Dadds, M.R., *et al.* "Imagery in human classical conditioning." *Psychological Bulletin* 122(1):89–103, 1997.

Davidson, J.R., *et al.* "Homeopathic treatment of depression and anxiety." *Alternative Therapy and Health Medicine* 3(1):46–49, 1997.

Davidson, R.J., *et al.* "Alterations in brain and immune function produced by mindfulness meditation." *Psychosomatic Medicine* 65(4):564–70, 2003.

M. Davis, E. Eshelman, and M. McKay. *The Relaxation & Stress Reduction Workbook*. Oakland, California: New Harbinger Publications, 2000.

Der, D.F., and P. Lewington. "Rational self-directed hypnotherapy: a treatment for panic attacks." *American Journal of Clinical Hypnosis* 32(3):160–67, 1990.

Ellis, A. *How to Make Yourself Happy and Remarkably Less Disturbable*. San Luis Obispo, California: Impact Publishers, 1999.

Ellis, A., and R. Harper. *A Guide to Rational Living*. North Hollywood, California: Wilshire Books, 1961.

Epstein, G. *Healing Visualizations Creating Health Through Imagery*. New York: Bantam Books, 1989.

Field, T., *et al.* "Job stress reduction therapies." *Alternative Therapy in Health and Medicine* 3(4):54–56, 1997.

Fried, R., & J. Grimaldi. *The Psychology and Physiology of Breathing*. New York: Plenum, 1993.

Gagne, E., and R.C. Toye. "The effects of therapeutic touch and relaxation therapy in reducing anxiety." *Archives of Psychiatric Nursing* 8(3):184–89, 1994.

Gerber, R. *Vibrational Medicine*. Santa Fe, New Mexico: Bear & Company, 1988.

Goodman, D. *Emotional Well-Being Through Rational Behavior*. Springfield, Illinois: Charles C. Thomas, 1978.

Howard, G.S., W.F. Nowlin, and M.J. Vargas. "Presurgical anxiety and postsurgical pain and adjustment: Effects of a stress innoculation procedure." *Clinical Psychology* 54(6):831–35.

Jacobson, E. *Progressive Relaxation*. Chicago: University of Chicago Press, 1938.

Laraia, M. "Panic disorder." *Advance for Nurse Practitioners* December 1995, pp. 24–29.

LeCron, L. *Self-Hypnosis*. New York: Signet, 1964.

Leibowitz, J., and B. Connington. *The Alexander Technique*. New York: Harper & Row, 1990.

London, R.T. "Strategies for treating PTSD." *Clinical Psychiatry News* 32(12):20, 2004.

Matsakis, A. *I Can't Get Over It: A Handbook for Trauma Survivors*. Oakland, California: New Harbinger Publications, Inc., 1992.

McKay, G.D., and D. Dinkmeyer. *How You Feel Is Up to You*. Atascadero, California: Impact Publishers, Inc., 1994.

Miller, J.J., K. Fletcher, and J. Kabat-Zinn. "Three-year follow-up and clinical implications of a mindfulness meditation-based stress reduction intervention in the treatment of anxiety disorders." *General Hospital Psychiatry* 17(3):192–200, 1995.

Moran, J.D. "Acupuncture and Chinese Medicine." In C.C. Clark, ed., *The Encyclopedia of Complementary Health Practice*. New York: Springer Publishing Company, 1999, pp. 281–88.

Pelletier, K. *Mind as Healer, Mind as Slayer*. New York: Doubleday, 1977.

———. *Sound Mind, Sound Body*. New York: Fireside, 1995.

———. *Stress Free for Good*. San Francisco: HarperSanFrancisco, 2005.

"Person-Centered Therapy." www.ed.utah.edu/psych/coursematerials/6200 Fall-02/6200.personcenteredtherapy.pdf. Accessed 5/14/05.

Redd, W.H., *et al.* "Fragrance administration to reduce anxiety during MR imaging." *Journal of Magnetic Resonance Imaging* 4(4):623–26, 1994.

Reiel, D.K., *et al.* "Mindfulness-based stress reduction and health-related quality of life in a heterogeneous patient population." *General Hospital Psychiatry* 23(4): 183–192, 2001.

Sabo, C.E., and S.R. Michael. "The influence of personal massage with music on anxiety and side effects associated with chemotherapy." *Cancer Nursing* 19(4):283–89, 1996.

Sachs, J. "A better way to treat depression and panic attacks: Nature's Prozac." *Let's Live* April 1997, pp. 42–43.

Sakai, M. "A clinical study of autogenic training-based behavioral treatment for panic disorder." *Pukuoka Igaku Zasshi* 87(3):77–84, 1996.

Salkovskis, P.M. "The cognitive approach to anxiety, threat beliefs, safety-seeking behavior, and the special case of health anxiety and obsessions." In Salkovskis, P.M., ed., *Frontiers of Cognitive Therapy*. New York: Guilford Press, 1996.

Serizawa, K. *Massage: The Oriental Method*. San Francisco: Japan Publications, 1972.

Simington, J.A., and G.P. Laing. "Effects of therapeutic touch on anxiety in the institutionalized elderly." *Clinical Nursing Research* 2(4):438–50, 1993.

Soulios, C., and B.J. Cox. "Brief treatment of emergency patients with panic attacks." *American Journal of Psychiatry* 7:944–46, 1992.

Splete, H. "CBT works across ethnicities." *Clinical Psychiatry News* 31(11):35, 2003.

Storz, D.R. "Getting a grip on anxiety." *The Clinical Advisor*, March 1999, pp. 17–26.

Weber, S. "The effects of relaxation exercises on anxiety levels in psychiatric inpatients." *Journal of Holistic Nursing* 14(3):196–205, 1996.

Wells, G.S., W.F. Nowlin, and M.J. Vargas. "Presurgical anxiety and postsurgical pain and adjustment." *Journal of Consulting and Clinical Psychology* 54(6):831–35, 1986.

Chapter 10 Relationships, Purpose, and Spirituality

Bourne, E.J. "Meaning, purpose, and spirituality," *The Anxiety and Phobia Workbook*. Oakland, California: New Harbinger Publications, 1995, pp. 379–96.

Burkhardt, M.A., and M.G. Nagai-Jacobson. "Spirituality and healing." In Barbara Montgomery Dossey, ed., *American Holistic Nurses' Associa-*

tion Core Curriculum for Holistic Nursing. Gaithersburg, Maryland: Aspen, 1997, pp. 42–51.

Caruba, A. "Worry your way to success: Ten secrets to successful problem solving plus where to find help." Maplewood, New Jersey: National Anxiety Center, 1992.

Cole, K.M. "Relaxation and dog visits in the CCU." *Nursing Clinics of North America* 30(3): 529–37, 1995.

Dadds, M.R., *et al.* "Prevention and early intervention for anxiety disorders: a controlled trial." *Journal of Consulting and Clinical Psychology* 65(4):627–35, 1997.

Gutman, D.A., and C.B. Nemeroff. "Persistent central nervous system effects of an adverse early environment: clinical and preclinical studies." *Physiological Behavior* 79(3):471–78.

Horrigan, B.J. "Spirituality and healthcare: A candid talk about possibilities." Interview with Leland R. Kaiser, Ph.D. *Explore: The Journal of Science and Healing* 1(1):49–56.

"How should I help myself and my family?" Washington, D.C.: American Psychological Association, 1996, p. 42.

Kortlander, E., P.C. Kendall, and S.M. Panicelli-Mindel. "Maternal expectations and attributions about coping in anxious children." *Journal of Anxiety Disorders* 11(3):297–315, 1997.

Fanning, P., and M. McKay. *Family Guide to Emotional Wellness.* Oakland, California: New Harbinger Publications, Inc., 2000.

"Role of family/impact on family." Portland State University, Research and Training Center on Family Support and Children's Mental Health, 1994.

Taylor, C.B., *et al.* "The effect of a home-based, case-managed, multifactorial risk-reduction program on reducing psychological distress in patients with cardiovascular disease." *Journal of Cardiopulmonary Rehabilitation* 17(3):157–62, 1997.

Chapter 11 Changes, Demands, Supports

Clark, C.C., ed. *The Encyclopedia of Complementary Health Practice.* New York: Springer, 1999.

Chapter 12 Finding and Working with the Right Practitioner

"Anxiety disorders: The role of psychotherapy in effective treatment." http://helping.apa.org/therapy/anxiety.html.

Bertakis, K.D., P. Franks, and R. Azari. "Effects of physician gender on patient satisfaction." *Journal of American Medical Womens Association* Spring 2003, pp. 69–75.

Boon, H., *et al.* "Visiting family physicians and naturopathic practitioners. Comparing patient-practitioner interactions." *Canadian Family Physician* 49:1481–87, 2003.

Clark, C.C., ed. *The Encyclopedia of Complementary Health Practice.* New York: Springer, 1999.

Cooper, L.A., *et al.* "Patient-centered communication, rating of care, and concordance of patient and physician race." *Annals of Internal Medicine* 139(11):907–915, 2003.

Flocke, S.A., W.L. Miller, and B.F. Crabtree. "Relationships between physician practice style, patient satisfaction, and attributes of primary care. *Journal of Family Practice* 51(10): 835–40, 2002.

Kinchen, K.S., *et al.* "Referral of patients to specialists: factors affecting choice of specialist by primary care physicians." *American Family Medicine* 2(3): 245–52, 2004.

Lazarus, A.A. *Mental Myths Revisited.* Atascadero, California: Impact Publishers, Inc., 2004.

Pinkerton, J.A., and H.A. Bush. "Nurse practitioners and physicians: patients' perceived health and satisfaction with care." *Journal of the American Academy of Nurse Practitioners* 12(6):211–17, 2000.

Pinniniti, N.R, N. Stolar, and S. Temple. "5-minute first aid for psychosis," *Current Psychiatry* 4(1), 36–48, 2005.

Rainer, S., R. Daughtridge, and P.D. Sloane. "Physician-patient communication in the primary care office: a systematic review. *Journal of the American Board of Family Practice* Vol. 15, 1:25–38, 2002.

Roter, D.L., *et al.* "Communication patterns of primary care physicians." *Journal of the American Medical Association* 277(4):350–56, 1997.

Roter, D.L., and J.A. Hall. "Physician gender and patient-centered communication: a critical review of empirical research." *Annual Review of Public Health* 25:497–519, 2004.

Street, R.L., Jr., *et al.* "Beliefs about control in the physician-patient relationship: effect on communication in medical encounters." *Journal of General Internal Medicine* 18(8):609–616, 2003.

Chapter 13 Putting It All Together: Your Anxiety Success Plan

HolisticHealth at Bellaonline.Com website. http://HolisticHealth.bellaonline.com.

McKay, G.D., and D. Dinkmeyer. *How You Feel Is Up to You: The Power of Emotional Choice.* Atascadero, California: Impact Publishers, Inc., 1994.

INDEX

WANT TO LIVE WELL?